OPIDEMIC
A Public Health Epidemic

by

J. Kimber Rotchford, M.D., M.P.H.

Copyright ©2018 OMS Ltd.

All rights reserved. No part of this book may be used or reproduced by any means, graphic, electronic, or mechanical, including photocopying, recording, taping, or by any information storage retrieval system without the written permission of the author except in the case of brief quotations embodied in critical articles and reviews.

This book expresses the views of J. Kimber Rotchford, M.D., M.P.H., a specialist in treating patients suffering from chronic pain and substance use disorders. He is a Fellow of the American College of Preventive Medicine and he is board certified in Public Health.

The book is published by Olympas Medical Services, Ltd. of Port Townsend, Washington. Printed in The United States of America.

First Edition 2018

Cover Art is reproduced from private collection of the author.
Front Cover: *Weeping Poppies* gift from artist Mary Ann Neale.
Back Cover: *James K Dragon* by Maggie Roe

ISBN-13: 978-1986794626
ISBN-10: 1986794628

Contact the Publisher
Olympas Medical Services
1136 Water St. Suite 107
Port Townsend, WA 98368

www.OPAS.us
staff@OPAS.us

This book can be ordered from Amazon and retail stores Purchasers of this book are invited to download a PDF copy with clickable links at: DrRotchford.com/guide

OPIDEMIC
A Public Health Epidemic

by

J. Kimber Rotchford, M.D., M.P.H.

OPIDEMIC
A Public Health Epidemic

J. Kimber Rotchford, M.D., M.P.H.

TABLE OF CONTENTS

Introduction	7

Chapter 1—Opidemic: An Opioid Abuse Epidemic	11
Basic Understanding of Addiction and Opioid Use Disorders	12
Addiction and Being Human—A Primer for the General Reader	13
Criteria to Establish the Diagnosis of Addiction	18
Criteria for Substance Abuse Are Not Commonly Appreciated	20
Treatment Options	23
Social and Community Responses	25
Cultural Influences on Substance Use Disorders	26
Puritan Heritage Affects Substance Use Disorders	32
Individualism	32
Policing Citizens' Behavior	34
Shame and Blame	36

Chapter 2—Myths and Misconceptions	38
Myth #1—We Know the Cause of Addiction	38
Myth #2—All Users Become Addicted	42
Myth #3—The Drug Causes the Addiction	44
Myth #4—Abstinence Is the Only Answer	46
Myth #5—Bad Doctors	46
Myth #6—Addicts Are Bad People	49

Chapter 3—Substance Abuse: A Public Health Concern   53
   a.) Background   53
   b.) What Has Been Our Approach?   54
   c.) Explanations for the Lack of a Public Health Response 55
   d.) Issues Specific to Opioids and Opioid Dependence   59
   e.) The Answer?   60
       Assuring Proper Medical Care   61
       Addressing Codependency   62
       Addressing Misbeliefs and Misunderstandings   63
   f.) Planning for Our Future   64

Chapter 4—Epidemics and Epidemiology   69
   a.) Definition of an Epidemic   69
   b.) What Epidemiologists Do   69
   c.) Do Statistics Lie?   71
   d.) The Interplay Between Facts and Beliefs   72
   e.) Complex Causes of Epidemics and Practical Implications 73
   f.) Complex Problems and Unintended Consequences   77
   g.) A Public Health Response Is Needed   79

Chapter 5—Agonist Therapy for Opioid Misuse   81
   a.) Definitions   81
   b.) Role of a Specialized Pain and Addiction Medical Practice 84
   c.) Treatment of Opioid Use Disorders Under DSM–V Criteria 87

Chapter 6—Medical Uses of Addictive Substances   **91**

   a.) General Principles   91

   b.) Issues Pertinent to Opioids   94

   c.) Issues with Benzodiazepines   97

   d.) Issues with Stimulants   98

   e.) Issues with Medical Cannabis   99

Appendix—Publications / Resources   **101**

   Publications—Recommended by Dr. Rotchford   101

   Handouts/References—On All Forms of SUDs   102

      Websites—Hosted by Dr. Rotchford   103

      Videos—Produced by Dr. Rotchford   103

      APPs—Developed by Dr. Rotchford   103

   Other Publications by J. Kimber Rotchford, M.D.   104

   About the Author   105

   About the Editors   106

Introduction

This compendium stems from a long-standing interest both in public health and addiction medicine. I was a health officer in rural Washington State more than thirty years ago. I then earned the designation of a Fellow of the American College of Preventive Medicine. An interest in addiction medicine also started early on in my medical career. Initially, the interest came from the number of general practice patients I cared for who had alcohol and tobacco use disorders. At that time there were also a few patients who were abusing pain pills. During the last 20 years, I have witnessed a serious plague of methamphetamine and opiate abuse. My response, in part, was to become one of the first physicians to be board certified in addiction medicine.

With my extended experience on the frontlines of attempting to better manage patients with opioid use disorders, I have wondered about the most effective prevention approaches. It is this wondering, coupled with a solid background in public health, which prompted me to write this compendium. The prevention of opiate use disorders and other substance use disorders is very complex, both medically as well as socially. Some even perceive the problem as being simply a function of spiritual or moral factors. With such complexity of causative factors, it is unlikely that simple solutions will resolve or mitigate the serious consequences of substance use disorders in America.

Opidemic—A Public Health Epidemic

In order to set the stage for potential preventive and therapeutic approaches, I start with a review of some of the basic medical understandings of opioid use disorders (OUDs) and addictions in general. I then explore some of the myths surrounding opioid abuse, the complex risk factors associated with OUDs, and effective treatment strategies for OUDS. The rest of the book lays out the foundations for a public health response, fortunately already underway in Washington State, but much progress is yet to come. Because epidemics have been best addressed by professionals within the public health arena, it makes sense that their leadership would be solicited in addressing the current opioid abuse epidemic.

As in a tuberculosis epidemic where a health officer would assure that effective treatment was readily available, I envision health departments and their associated public health professionals and institutions taking a confirmed leadership role. The public health community has the expertise to assure a comprehensive and evidence-based approach. It also has the expertise to better secure collaborative efforts by various providers within a community. Public health currently lacks the financial and the clinical expertise. This is true both in most urban as well as rural communities. It also lacks a tradition of dealing with non-infectious epidemics. It did, however, effectively address the AIDS epidemic. To achieve this, it had to educate and attempt to change behavior regarding IV drug use and sexual behavior. Having an OUD is similar to having AIDS. Both diseases cannot be cured, but they can be effectively managed by a combination of medical as well as behavioral interventions. Public health consequently has a recent history of successfully curbing epidemics similar to the opioid misuse epidemic. Given proper funding and authority, I am confident public health would effectively manage the opioid crisis and achieve effective prevention strategies.

Recently, I learned that the Seattle Health Department has a grant to assure that Medication Assisted Treatment (MAT) is readily available for all who suffer with opioid use disorders. They even have policies in place to assure patients receive MAT, even when abusing other substances such as alcohol. This is a harm reduction model, and this model has a longstanding track record in curbing the consequences from most epidemics. It is the rare exception where the vector(s) of an infectious disease epidemic can be entirely eradicated. This is particularly true with TB epidemics and other infectious disease epidemics where relatively low prevalence rates become the objective. Similarly, we cannot entirely eliminate addictive substances (the vector of SUDs). Chapter 6 outlines the essential role of addictive substances in modern medicine.

As a health officer, I also recall in the 1980s reading chest x-rays in patients who had been diagnosed with TB. As the health officer, I was able to assure patients who suffered from TB received effective treatment, whether through the health department or through community providers. I am passionate about making our American response to the opioid epidemic similar to successful efforts to manage past epidemics, such as with TB, polio, and AIDS epidemics.

The compendium has six chapters with associated links. The first two chapters provide some basics for understanding the opioid epidemic, along with common misunderstandings. The next chapter, brings us to solutions through the help of an empowered public health response. The following chapters are intended to give further background information regarding public health and clinical information. A primer for an informed public health response to an epidemic, epidemiology, is provided in chapter 4. In the final chapters, I've supplied more detailed information regarding Medication Assisted Treatment (MAT) in the care for opioid use disorders and lastly, as already mentioned, a brief discussion of the essential role of addictive substances in medical care.

Chapter 1—*Opidemic: An Opioid Abuse Epidemic*

"Opidemic" is a term coined to describe the significant morbidity and mortality associated with the recent upsurge of opioid use and abuse in the United States. It is a combination of the words opioid and epidemic to accentuate the disease's uniqueness and severity. The Opidemic phenomenon has become widely accepted in the United States as an epidemic. Let us address the Opidemic as we have done effectively with other epidemics such as tuberculosis, influenza, and heart disease. The best response to a serious epidemic is to use the professionals with a proven track record of managing epidemics: our public health professionals.

Opioid use disorder (opioid addiction) is a biological disease. It is in the family of substance use disorders (SUDs). This compendium introduces the complex and multifactorial nature of opioid abuse and associated epidemics. Associated loss and suffering from opioid misuse extends to the entire community. The costs from this poorly contained disease extend well beyond direct individual and medical costs. Schools (substandard learning and behavior), businesses (compromised work), the criminal justice system (police, courts, prisons), social services, and the budgets of the federal and local governments are all seriously impacted by the Opidemic.

Public health expertise makes it the ideal means to map out and coordinate an effective response to any epidemic. Formal estimates of savings from effective prevention and care are in the range of 7-12 times the money invested. However, to properly and effectively apply a public health intervention, it is helpful to understand not only addiction, specifically opioid use disorder and its medically indicated treatments, but also the barriers that have had an impact on implementing an effective approach to this now widespread epidemic. In the next few chapters, I attempt to clarify definitions, remove assumptions, and contend with pertinent biases, myths, and cultural factors.

Basic Understanding of Addiction and Opioid Use Disorders

A recent survey found that both average adults and primary care physicians in the United States cling to a variety of misperceptions and stereotypes about opioid addiction.[1] The survey revealed some surprising knowledge deficits among both the public and healthcare providers. That

---

[1] https://neuropathyandhiv.blogspot.com/2013/07/understanding-opioid-addiction.html#.WqyHVejwZPY

many doctors misunderstand key facets of opioid abuse was substantiated in another 2015 survey.[2]

As the above surveys indicate, there remains much ignorance around opioid addiction. What immediately follows provides only a basic and brief introduction to opioid use disorders and addiction. In Chapter 5 (Agonist Therapy for Opioid Use Disorders) and Chapter 6 (Medical Uses of Addictive Substances), the reader can find more detailed material concerning some of our medical understandings and clinical principles as they relate to the management of substance use disorders, including opioid use disorders.

Addiction and Being Human—A Primer for the General Reader[3]

The heading, "Addiction and Being Human," hopes to mitigate cultural shaming and prejudices directed toward those who struggle with addictions. The concept of addiction may mean something different

---

[2] https://www.jhsph.edu/news/news-releases/2015/survey-many-doctors-misunderstand-key-facets-of-opioid-abuse.html

[3] The discussion "Addiction and Being Human" was a public presentation at St. Paul's Episcopal Church in Port Townsend, Washington on July 26th 2017. In this compendium, some of its contents were utilized as a primer for the general reader for issues related to substance use disorders and in particular opioid use disorders.

depending on the context. For the purposes herein, we use the current medical term for addiction: a substance use disorder. A better appreciation of the nature of substance use disorders—and how we think about them—will provide more insight into how to approach the subject with care and tact.

More than any other chronic disease that afflicts us, such as diabetes, tuberculosis, and other mental health disorders, our susceptibility to substance use disorders is consistent with a universal and fundamental attribute of human nature. The substances associated with substance use disorders "hijack" parts of the brain designed to promote higher forms of learning and remembering. The capacity to learn and remember clearly represent essential human attributes. While we most often give homage to our conscious thinking, subconscious mechanisms conceivably dominate human behavior and our basic perceptions. In brief, addictive substances affect the same areas of the brain which allow us to both consciously and subconsciously learn and remember.

While the mechanisms involved with learning and remembering have been "hijacked," people with addictions are not stupid! Indeed, they learn well. One could say that, in some ways, they learn too well. All individuals find it challenging to entirely forget what is no longer of use or problematic. An ease at learning complex patterns subconsciously, as we see in excellent athletes and performers, involves circuits in the brain involved with addictions. An ease at learning complex patterns, particularly subconsciously, is arguably a serious and unappreciated risk factor for developing a substance use disorder.

Why are substance use disorders considered chronic and incurable diseases? The simplest answer may be as already noted: it is challenging and perhaps impossible for humans to entirely forget what they have learned. Remnants of memories and experiences, whether conscious or not, seem to remain in intact brains. A second explanation, consistent with the first, is that receptors on brain cells and neural circuits are permanently affected by addictive substances. Evidence for long-term changes are supported by PET scans of the brain. Even five years or so after past use of cocaine, subconscious circuits light up with proper cues. This occurs despite no conscious awareness by the individual who is being examined.

In addition to these and other objective brain changes caused by addictive substances, the best support for using the medical model to treat addiction is evidence that when substance use disorders are addressed as a disease the outcomes improve. With complex issues that are incompletely understood, it is best to be pragmatic. From a pragmatic standpoint, the medical model is the optimal method to achieve the most cost-effective outcomes for substance use disorders.

In addition to promoting effective medical approaches, a robust public health response incorporates system approaches. Our historical emphasis on using will power, shame, regulation, prohibition, and the criminal justice system as our primary and sometimes only tools has had limited results and has presumably aggravated the problem. A familiarity with cultural influences is essential to better understand the hows and whys behind varied responses to substance abuse. The American culture itself has had a significant impact on the prevention, recognition, and effective care of substance use disorders.

The suffering and the premature deaths associated with substance use disorders are of staggering magnitude. They arguably represent our greatest public health threat.[4] As with tuberculosis, it is unlikely that substance use disorders will be totally eradicated. Addictive substances are going to be around. They are not only appealing but also often quite helpful. They can be essential tools in modern medical care. Lastly, human brains and behavior are not likely to rapidly and significantly change.

The physiological mechanisms and genetics associated with substance use disorders are perhaps better understood than most common diseases. However, as with most diseases, why one patient is more susceptible, and why some people do better than others, with or without appropriate treatment, are questions with unclear answers. Understanding addictions is complex, both socially and with individuals. Simple reductionist models are unlikely to reflect common findings.

With tuberculosis, which generated the Koch postulates for identifying an infectious causal agent, we know that exposure to the

---

[4] See further discussion in Chapter 4

tuberculosis bacteria is required. Questions remain, however, as to why some people get the disease following exposure and others not? Furthermore, why do some people respond to standard therapies and others not? We understand bacterial resistance, but this does not entirely explain the variability in responses. We know that socioeconomic factors, immune status, and comorbid medical conditions also play a role. So, even with the infectious disease tuberculosis, which promulgated scientific criteria for causality, there remain many unknown and confounding variables related to the incidence and prevalence of tuberculosis. In addition, despite dramatic strides in our understanding and treatment of tuberculosis, tuberculosis still remains a significant public health threat.

In addressing the opioid epidemic, it is reasonable to employ the same principles for understanding and responding to tuberculosis and other infectious epidemics. To best respond to a disease such as tuberculosis, one must be able to diagnose it. How do physicians make the diagnosis of a substance use disorder? Unfortunately, as of yet there are no specific biomarkers like those we associate with tuberculosis or diabetes. However, this lack of a biomarker doesn't mean that opioid use disorders do not reflect disease as it is commonly defined. The changes in the brain associated with substance use disorders are quite objective. Furthermore, there are valid and reliable criteria to establish the diagnosis, and validated questionnaires exist which allow clinicians to reliably make a diagnosis.

When severe substance use disorders (SUDs) are often obvious to family and friends, the disease is still frequently denied by the patient. Is this lack of recognition of the disease, often called denial, a product of brains not working properly, or would it be closer to the truth to attribute the denial to cultural factors or subconscious psychological factors? No clear-cut answers can be readily found. Nonetheless, cultural or social denial is one thing and individual denial is another.

Criteria to Establish the Diagnosis of Addiction

Many formal and reliable criteria are used to establish the diagnosis of addiction or substance use disorders. The following are current criteria based on evidence and expertise. As an example, they relate to opioid use disorders.

An opioid use disorder is a problematic pattern of opioid use leading to clinically significant impairment or distress, as manifested by at least two of the following, occurring within a 12-month period:

1. Opioids are often taken in larger amounts or over a longer period than was intended.

2. There is a persistent desire or unsuccessful efforts to cut down or control opioid use.

3. A great deal of time is spent in activities necessary to obtain the opioid, use the opioid, or recover from its effects.

4. Craving, or a strong desire or urge, to use opioids.

5. Recurrent opioid use resulting in a failure to fulfill major role obligations at work, school, or home.

6. Continued opioid use despite having persistent or recurrent social or interpersonal problems caused or exacerbated by the effects of opioids.

7. Important social, occupational, or recreational activities are given up or reduced because of opioid use.

8. Recurrent opioid use in situations in which it is physically hazardous.

9. Continued opioid use despite knowledge of having a persistent or recurrent physical or psychological problem that is likely to have been caused or exacerbated by the substance.

10. Tolerance, as defined by either of the following: a.) a need for markedly increased amounts of opioids to achieve intoxication or desired effect; or b.) a markedly diminished effect with continued use of the same amount of an opioid. Note: this criterion is not considered to be met for those taking opioids solely under appropriate medical supervision.

11. Withdrawal, as manifested by either of the following: a.) the characteristic opioid withdrawal syndrome or b.) opioids (or a closely related substance) are taken to relieve or avoid withdrawal symptoms.

Criteria for Substance Abuse Are Not Commonly Appreciated

1. No current signs or symptoms are required. The criteria pertain to *any* 12-month period, whether past or present.
2. No single criteria makes the diagnosis, and the lack of any one criteria is not diagnostic.
3. Because it takes having two criteria to make the diagnosis and criteria 10 and 11, which reflect physical dependence are just two of the 11 criteria, one can have the disease and not have symptoms of withdrawal or tolerance (physical dependence), whether current or in the past. For example, cannabis use disorders occur in about 15% of regular users, but cannabis use disorders are not commonly associated with signs or symptoms of significant physical dependence and withdrawal. Perhaps as few as 15% of patients with cannabis use disorders show apparent signs of physical dependence. Conversely, some antidepressants and blood pressure medicines can induce serious withdrawal symptoms, but are not addictive substances. It takes at least two of the criteria to be met to consider the possibility of a mild substance use disorder.
4. One doesn't have to break any laws, be unethical, or morally deficient to have a substance use disorder.
5. One does not need to want to use or want to continue to use the substance to have a substance use disorder. Conversely, not liking

or wanting to use the substance doesn't exclude having a substance use disorder.

6. The diagnosis does not depend on whether the opioid was a prescription, how it was used, obtained, or what dose used. These aspects can be, however, risk factors for developing or having the disease.

7. As with most chronic diseases, particularly those that affect the brain, the disease has a continuum of severity from mild to severe disease. SUDs often wax and wane, and no set of criteria are universal or specific to everyone.

8. Frequency of use or duration of use are only relevant if duration is longer than was intended.

The brain adaptations and pathophysiology associated with substance use disorders are complex, diffuse, and much knowledge is yet to be gained. They vary significantly from one abused substance to another. What we seem to know most about is the area of the brain that is initially "hijacked" by substances of abuse. This area of the brain is called the reward center and its headquarters is the nucleus accumbens. It is this area of the brain that allows us to learn complex tasks and to predict further reward, or lack thereof. Indeed, the nucleus accumbens could be described as the main processor for the way it relates to higher forms of learning. As already mentioned, learning and remembering are emblematic of what it is to be human. Substance use disorders, as they reflect dysfunctional learning and remembering, characterize a basic human susceptibility to substance use disorders, as well as other forms of addiction.

What happens normally in the nucleus accumbens to promote healthy learning is quite similar to what happens when an addictive substance is used. As far as we know, all forms of higher learning, all substance use disorders, and some behaviors such as gambling, sex, and pain behavior all start with surges of dopamine in the nucleus accumbens. A substance which directly causes a significant dopamine surge in the nucleus accumbens is hence addictive. When a dopamine surge does not occur with exposure, then technically the substance is not an addictive substance. Substances that do not directly cause a release of dopamine may be readily abused, though technically they are not addictive substances. An example of such substances might be LSD or other hallucinogens.

Substances or behaviors associated with higher surges in dopamine are more addictive. Substances associated with less dramatic surges in dopamine might, in susceptible individuals, still induce a substance use disorder. Cannabis and refined sugars are examples of substances with significantly less dramatic dopamine surges. Heroin, nicotine, and methamphetamine are examples of substances which result in higher surges of dopamine. Hence, these latter substances are among the most addictive. The intensity of the surge in dopamine in the nucleus accumbens remains the best predictor of a substance's or a behavior's addiction potential.

Fortunately, even with highly addictive substances such as heroin, most people will not develop an addiction with occasional use. Only 20% of the Vietnam War veterans who experimented with heroin eventually developed an opioid use disorder. As with most learned behavior, addictive behavior and substance use must be repeated for the disease to develop. Based on physiological mechanisms involved, it is assumed that a contingency is required, as is true with most forms of higher learning. Therefore, the concept of cues and triggers, and their subsequent management, play essential roles in addiction recovery.

Note, no evidence suggests that the brain responds to an addictive substance based on whether the substance is legal, prescribed, or used as a food or not. There are, however, many established, contextual variables, such as related mental health conditions and genetics that contribute to the susceptibility for developing a substance use disorder, its management, and its prognosis.

Treatment Options

In general, substance use disorders are best managed in an individualized manner. A combination of medical as well as behavioral interventions which include family and community support are associated with good outcomes. In further topics, we explore other effective treatments. It is worth noting here as an important treatment principle: **the best single predictor for a good outcome remains the time in treatment.**

Time in treatment is such a good predictor, because substance use disorders are chronic, relapsing disorders. As with most major mental health disorders and commonly addressed medical conditions, such as diabetes and heart disease, care of SUDs is chronic and often lifelong. The benefit of combining treatment approaches in SUDs is no different than with most chronic diseases such as diabetes, heart disease, arthritis, or depression.

Substance use disorders associated with alcohol, stimulants, and sedatives are most often addressed through behavioral means and total abstinence. Even with a valid emphasis on abstinence, as is the case with alcohol use disorders, many medicines are FDA approved for alcohol use disorders. These medicines have been proven to help some patients to achieve sobriety and provide harm reduction.

Medication Assisted Treatment (MAT) in opioid use disorders, whether with methadone or buprenorphine, has substantial supporting evidence. In some studies, when moderate to severe opioid use disorders exist, the annual mortality rate alone is 4 to 5 times greater with abstinence-based approaches as compared to medication supported approaches. Patients who have more serious opioid use disorders and succeed at remaining abstinent seem to have more stress-related medical conditions, painful conditions, and shorter and less fulfilling lives than their counterparts who are managed with MAT. The need for MAT with an opioid use disorder is hence distinctly different than from alcohol use disorders. In alcohol use disorders, abstinence is a good and reliable surrogate marker for a robust recovery and future well-being. In contrast, abstinence with moderate to severe opioid use disorders is a relatively poor predictor of a favorable outcome, albeit abstinence is still commonly encouraged. Even the Washington State Pain Rules, designed to limit opioid prescribing, acknowledge that prognosis is poor without agonist therapy (MAT) in moderate to severe opioid use disorders.

Social and Community Responses

A comprehensive, systematic approach that addresses both individual rights and the larger community needs is warranted. This approach would assure ready access to necessary medical care. This approach would minimize the current social and financial consequences of substance misuse and emphasize appropriate compassion to better assure effective medical care and outcomes. Prohibition and adversarial approaches consistent with our regulatory and criminal justice strategies are not working and are unlikely to play a major role in any long-term, effective approach. Placing blame on individuals and other adversarial approaches are to be transformed into collaborative efforts. It warrants repetition: substance use disorders are diseases and the epidemics associated with same merit public health expertise.

In addition to our inherited physiology, human nature is such that we behave and perceive based on our individual and social conditioning. At times, human conditioning and physiology can be so dominant they result in someone doing the opposite of what they intended or decided to do. To better assure that collective values are honored, we need experts who can help us modify our counterproductive behavior and beliefs. In so doing, improved personal and public health can be expected. Perhaps substance use disorders, more than any other ailment, remind us that on a personal as well as a cultural basis we are subject to conditioning. We as humans sometimes learn *too well* and have problems forgetting.

Cultural Influences on Substance Use Disorders

Cultural influences as well as individual experiences are important to appreciate in understanding a better response to opioid use disorders. Like diabetes and other chronic diseases, when dealing effectively with opioid use disorders, we must treat not only biological and behavioral factors but also remain sensitive to contributing cultural factors. The significantly high prevalence of substance use related problems in the United States demands explanations that encompass not only the biological but the cultural factors as well. Once these cultural and biological mechanisms that promote opioid abuse are better appreciated, we are better prepared to effectively establish a comprehensive public health intervention and, ultimately, an effective prevention strategy.

People who suffer from addictive processes are commonly predisposed to denial, blame, and shame of themselves and others. In startling ways, the self-destructive patterns associated with addictions often continue despite the serious consequences. But should the behavior be such a surprise given what we know? When people or cultures perseverate in behaviors that were once helpful, but are now dysfunctional, they exhibit commonly observed neurotic behavior. Addictive processes are at the more extreme end of these common neurotic processes. In the case of addictive processes associated with substance use, significant brain pathology (objective changes in brain tissue) is routinely found, which also helps explain the significant and dysfunctional behaviors observed.

While neurotic and addictive patterns are common human attributes, the question remains: why is the prevalence of addictions in the United States seemingly so high? The answers are complex and multifactorial. Some are listed below without an attempt to prioritize their relative importance. All cultures have similar factors. It is perhaps the excess of these factors that may help explain the American predisposition to addictive disorders.

Availability and access to substances of abuse are important and proven contributors and risk factors to help explain the development of substance use disorders. It makes sense, for if one does not have the opportunity to be exposed repeatedly to a substance, it becomes impossible to become addicted.

Eliminating easy access has been the primary thrust of our preventive approaches as exemplified in the "War on Drugs" and the unprecedented powers provided to the DEA. This approach, while having some merit, does little to paint the entire picture.[5]

The concept of codependence, while somewhat abstract, is useful. It commonly comes up in recovery from addictions. It is considered a significant risk factor for all substance use disorders. Codependency can be defined in many possible ways. A useful definition is that codependency is an attribute of people who tend to have a high emotional charge vis a vis their responsibility to manage the feelings and behavior of others. Many of us have grown up with parents or loved ones who have said things like: "You make me so proud;" "You make me so angry;" or "You make me feel ashamed." From caring authority figures, these sorts of comments can readily condition children to feel responsible for how others feel.

Is American culture more codependent than other cultures? Americans do tend to use intimidation and force to control the behavior of others. Since one's behavior often reflects underlying feelings and beliefs, using force to control another's behavior, outside the context of self-defense, may reflect attributes of codependence. The use of intimidation and force is prominent and reflected through our laws, police, prisons, penalties, shaming, isolation from others, military might, religious determinants, or other effective means of control. These means of force are not limited to governmental entities. Parents, spouses,

---

[5] http://www.drugpolicy.org/issues/brief-history-drug-war

institutions, and others in authority often feel justified to use heavy-handed means of intimidation and control.

It is sometimes necessary to put limits to dysfunctional behavior, and such limits may reflect healthy compassion. By healthy compassion, I refer to the human capacity to respond to other living things through empathy and with concern for their well-being. It is encapsulated in the great commandment of loving your neighbor as yourself. Healthy compassion may lead one to intervene, whether gently or more forcefully. Even professionals confuse compassion with codependence. Some physicians have been criticized for being too compassionate in their prescribing of pain medicines. I maintain that a physician can never be *too* compassionate. That is, a physician cannot be too empathetic or concerned about a patient's well-being. But physicians can be too codependent and, in so doing, contribute to a patient's and their communities' ill health. An example of this would be a doctor refilling a prescription simply to help the patient feel better at the time, rather than be attentive to the appropriate indications or long-term risks and benefits for the patient and their community.

The question of being over-attentive to the feelings and behavior of others comes up routinely with parents. What is a parent's responsibility in relation to managing and controlling the behavior and feelings of one's baby or child? Responding appropriately to a child's feelings or limiting their problematic behavior is quite appropriate and may even be life sustaining. At a certain point, however, attempts to control or feel responsible for the feelings of child is dysfunctional. At what age? It seems to differ even from one child to the next. Similarly, it can be challenging to define where compassion and concern for your neighbor translates into codependence. Nonetheless, the distinction is valid and clinically important.

How might the charitable attributes of the American culture and its concern for others be distinguished from attributes of codependence? Many contextual variables apply, but when one is prepared to identify codependent behavior, it becomes more obvious. As with parents, equivocal answers pertain to the question of when one should stop attempting to control or feel responsible for the feelings and behavior of a child. Nonetheless, while some behavior is ambiguous and must be judged by context, it remains true that overprotective behavior is often counterproductive.

For better and for worse, America's military strength has been described as the police force of the world.[6] American police seem prone to use undue force.[7] What is the basis for this inclination to feel responsible for controlling unwanted behavior? Within our own society, is it related to burgeoning laws and regulations? In any event, the extent of these control efforts has many concerned. I argue they reflect, at least

---

[6] https://www.usnews.com/news/articles/2016-09-16/the-us-is-the-worlds-police-force

[7] Wikipedia - The Use of Force
https://en.wikipedia.org/wiki/Use_of_force#U.S._statistics

in part, the American predisposition towards codependence and with it an inclination to fear what one cannot control.

Illusions of control are typical among those suffering with addictive disorders as well as in the larger American culture. Prohibition, more laws, stiffer penalties, more money, more research, larger defense budget, or predetermined knowledge of God's will are just some of the means of feeling in control over real or imagined threats. While important steps must be undertaken to control any epidemic, it is helpful to avoid illusions of control. Only a handful of the epidemics related to infectious diseases have resulted in everlasting control or total elimination of the vector(s). For the most part, particularly when epidemics are multifactorial and are related to basic human nature and biology, the best outcomes are achieved when harm reduction strategies are used. This is why effective public health strategies are commonly labelled as harm reduction strategies. Attempts to over control or regulate a force of nature can be counterproductive as one could argue was the case with the "War on Drugs."

The *Drug Policy Alliance* is an organization of people committed to reassessing our need to control the use of drugs. Such efforts have had significant influence in changing the laws as they relate to marijuana. As the effect on liberalization of marijuana laws become acknowledged, we might expect similar changes related to all substances of abuse. While an absence of laws or rules related to substances of abuse is not reasonable, throughout history the pendulums of change often swing from one extreme to the other. Perhaps only then is a better balance eventually established?

Puritan Heritage Affects Substance Use Disorders

Puritanical beliefs justified and promoted punishment and penance for bad behavior. Despite some exceptions, jails and prisons are still not designed to be rehabilitative. They impart justice and punishment. Some of our prisons are still called "penitentiaries." It is well beyond the scope of this paper to fully explore the benefits and harm of punitive approaches to human behavior. When bad behavior stems from unhealthy brains, it very probable that better behavior will ensue from efforts to help brains heal, rather than through imposing further stress, shame, and blame.

Mental illness and substance use disorders can physically damage brains and their proper functioning. Social conditioning can also promote dysfunctional behaviors. Flawed judgement, faulty insights, or socially unacceptable behavior predictably ensue. These facts put into question the justice of punishing behaviors over which the victims have little control. Indeed, the disease of addiction, perhaps more than any human understanding, puts into question common beliefs about free will.

Individualism

Individualism is another American attribute contributing to addictive disorders. The story of the heroic pioneer man comes to mind. Our country was founded by these highly individualistic pioneers who carved out their own livelihoods and land, initiating the idealism of the "American dream." But, individualism can make it problematic to accept the "we" so prominent in the first step of any 12-step program. It becomes challenging for someone highly individualistic to appreciate how the "we" of the first step translates into a more functional "I." Americans readily believe the corollary: "If I help the *I*, the *we* benefits." There is some truth in this, and political tensions often arise around opposing beliefs in these matters. Nonetheless, from a pragmatic standpoint, an important step in confronting codependence and an inclination for using force is to remember the "we" and "our" approach.

In sporting events, business, education, and so many other endeavors, it is motivation, persistence, and a confidence in what one can and must do that often translates into better results. In other matters, however, the approach of individualism and self-will may be destructive, and most often is not part of a sustainable solution. On this subject of the "we" versus the "I" approach, paradoxically, the "closed" communities of drug and alcohol abusers are potent sources of support. This social support, as dysfunctional as it may be, likely mitigates the stress not only from having the disease and its repercussions, but also limits the consequences of individualism and isolation.

In the past, rugged individualism in America was antidoted by religious institutions, which promoted a collective approach for salvation and life. There was an acknowledged dependence on a loving and just God—"Let God be the judge!" "In God We Trust" is printed on

American money, but given the prevalence of individualism, it is now a relatively rare American who takes this powerful American adage to heart.

Individualism can progress into egocentricity and lack of openness. In the discussion of solutions or responses to the Opidemic, one rarely hears: "What do other countries and cultures do? How successful are they?" In being "addicted" to the American way, Americans are at odds with seeking outside input or perspectives. The same patterns are commonly encountered in patients who are addicted. At the point when a patient becomes open to receiving outside input and the process of asking for help is encouraged and experienced, the patient's prognosis is greatly improved.

Policing Citizens' Behavior

For better or for worse, the United States government takes on the role of policing citizens' behavior, even when the behavior is the result of physiological processes beyond the control of a person, as is the case in those suffering from a serious substance use disorder. People with addictions are criminalized, marginalized, and shamed. People addicted to substances or other addictive behaviors are highly discriminated against. The majority of people in American jails are there for mental health and substance abuse related crimes. In treating these individuals as criminals, it only further adds to the discrimination, distrust, and misunderstandings. The "War on Drugs" often translate into an "us and them" perception rather than "we" or team approaches. Our cultural inclination to battle or make war against behaviors we object to likely reflects a deep-rooted cultural contributor to substance abuse.

In the United States there has been a longstanding history of control efforts through laws and regulations. It has been less than 100 years since we attempted to prohibit alcohol abuse through a constitutional amendment. In relation to substances of abuse, the United States is arguably the most regulated society. The Drug Enforcement Agency (DEA) has been given powers second only to the Internal Revenue Service (IRS). The results of such power and control efforts are nonetheless associated with a gross failure to control the abuse of substances. One epidemic after another rises, sometimes even in the same class of substances abused (eg: prescription drug abuse, then heroin abuse, and now fentanyl like drug abuse).

A simple association between a failed outcome and our highly regulatory approach does not demonstrate causation. Of course, many factors remain at play. Nonetheless, it is worth noting that the paradoxical and seemingly counterproductive acceptance of being powerless works for many who suffer from addictions. Might this approach be more effective as a society? Based on human nature and evidence from countries with less substance abuse, it is likely that less regulated drug use and decriminalization—as well as managing substance abuse through a robust public health approach—would have better outcomes.[8]

Shame and Blame

People with addictions are often shamed and blamed. Even patients on prescribed pain medications for chronic issues can experience significant prejudices in medical settings—to the point of undue suffering and death. People with addictions commonly confront challenges to obtain proper and adequate medical care. It is arguably the case that prejudices and biases associated with addiction are comparable to those encountered with race or sexual preferences. In addition, overlap occurs with some examples of racism. Not uncommonly some people will justify their racist attitudes based on addictive behavior. For instance, many have defended racism towards Native Americans by pigeonholing them as alcoholics; as well, the stereotyped use of cocaine and marijuana by African Americans has likely fueled racist attitudes.

Government officials and institutional policies support a "Just say no" approach to kicking addictions. This approach assumes that the answer to addiction is more willpower, discipline, and perseverance, as in the self-sufficient pioneer man. It is also commensurate with some religious beliefs: that salvation is achieved through the ability to control one's own sinful nature and that of others. This approach demoralizes

---

[8] Drug Decriminalization in Portugal: Lessons for Creating Fair and Successful Drug Policies https://papers.ssrn.com/sol3/papers.cfm?abstract_id=1464837

the individual with shame and blame and fails to acknowledge substance abuse as a disease. While partially preventable like most infectious diseases, substance use disorders do not warrant condemnation for those affected by them.

Chapter 2—Myths and Misconceptions

We have already discussed above the survey which demonstrated ignorance about opioid use disorders, even among professionals. We have delved into cultural and social factors that influence our attitudes. Facts and critical thinking often do not compete well with beliefs. When it comes to human behavior and politics, beliefs inevitably trump the facts. Nonetheless, the list of common myths and misunderstandings regarding substance use disorders—and attempts to explain, prevent, and respond to the Opidemic—is provided as a way to counter some of the widespread ignorance and fear.

Myth #1—We Know the Cause of Addiction

Many explanations exist regarding the common misconception that we know the cause of addiction. Established risk factors or factors highly associated with the Opidemic are not causal. In other words, the causation pattern is not one of "If A then B." This "If A then B" assumption is perhaps the most important lapse in critical thinking as it relates to understanding and better responding to the Opidemic. It is a variant of the *post hoc ergo propter hoc* fallacy. It simply states that if something occurs after something else, the preceding event is the cause. Based on common human experience, we tend to assume that what precedes an event is likely to have caused it. This assumption is not always supported by critical or scientific thinking. We know that attributing causation is much more complex than identifying preceding or associated events. We often can only appreciate risk factors and do our best to reduce same. Let us review three examples of the *post hoc ergo propter hoc* fallacy as it relates to the Opidemic and addictions.

Example 1: Patients who are prescribed higher doses of opioids, particularly methadone, are more likely to die of an overdose. The fallacy is to assume that it is simply the higher dose of prescribed opioid that caused the death. When one looks closer at the facts, we find many lives are saved, a much greater number than those dying, when high dose opioids are properly used. It's not the dose, but the improper selection, monitoring, support, and care for comorbid conditions, let alone other substances abused, that best explain the mortality rates associated with higher doses of opioids. Further evidence supports the fallacy of assuming that higher doses best explain the overdose rates. In Washington State, based on its Prescription Monitoring Program data, no sound correlation exists between the total amount of opiates prescribed in a county and its number of overdose deaths.

Common sense also supports the notion that sicker patients are more likely to have more complications and higher mortality. Patients who require higher doses of opioids are likely more ill for a host of reasons and, because of the severity of their illness, more likely to experience greater mortality. For example, patients on higher doses of insulin are more likely to die from an overdose or have other complications. It is not a coincidence that a disproportionate number of overdose deaths occur in Medicaid patients. Among other confounding variables, patients on Medicaid are commonly more ill and disabled. They often have co-occurring disorders. To attribute the death of these patients simply to higher doses is fallacious.

Example 2: Another example of the *post hoc ergo propter hoc* fallacy stems from the belief that patients who develop heroin addiction often started with the use or abuse of prescription painkillers and, hence, the reason given for the heroin epidemic is the over-prescribing of opioids for pain. While the prevalence of a substance in an environment is an established risk factor for abuse of the substance, to explain heroin addiction primarily on doctors' prescribing is a classic *post hoc ergo propter hoc* fallacy. Heroin addiction has been a problem long before doctors started prescribing opiates more readily. Increased laxity in prescribing opioids occurred in the 1990s when pain started to be considered the 5th vital sign.

Other explanations are more likely to account for the increase of heroin addiction, such as the upsurge in access to heroin, coupled with plummeting costs, which soared after the United States' invasion of Afghanistan. The invasion is known to have increased the production and distribution of heroin. In addition, as pain practitioners have lost their licenses and many criminalized,[9] there is a common upswing in demand for heroin in the community. This seems to counter the argument that bad prescribers are the reason for heroin abuse and complications. The propensity for opioid use disorders is in significant part genetic, and significant risk factors, aside from a history of using a pain prescription, are involved. From an epidemiological standpoint, these other factors are much more likely to explain the risk of development of the disease or complications from its use.

In Washington State, as physicians have been prescribing less opioids, the overdose rate from prescription drugs has predictably gone down since it is only through prescriptions that prescription drugs are circulated or abused. Meanwhile, the rate of heroin overdoses has skyrocketed. Overdose deaths related to heroin have always dwarfed the rate associated with prescription overdoses. Nonetheless, the regulatory emphasis has been on blaming "unprofessional" and/or "overly compassionate" licensed physicians.[10]

Example 3: Risk factors are often attributed as primary causes. However, just because Monday mornings are associated with a higher frequency of heart attacks does not mean that the primary cause for heart attacks is a Monday morning! While the stress of Monday morning, for a host of reasons, may be a factor, to ascribe Monday morning as causal is

---

[9] Libby RT, *The Criminalization of Medicine - America's War on Doctors*, Praeger Series on Contemporary Health and Living, Westport, Connecticut, 2008 210pgs.

[10] www.doctorsofcourage.org was established for and by physicians unjustly and without due process subjected to DEA enforcement efforts.

ludicrous. But we often make similar causative accusations regarding opioid overdoses. Understandably, some factors might aggravate the likelihood of an overdose. Like Monday mornings, they must not be assumed to be causative, at least not in the normal sense of the word.

Myth #2—All Users Become Addicted

As discussed above, the notion of causation in medicine and public health can be confusing and often poorly understood. Using the traditional Koch's postulates, one can be comfortable attributing the cause of the disease of tuberculosis to the tuberculosis bacilli. We readily accept that the disease originates with a gram-negative rod belonging to the family of mycobacterium. Nonetheless, some people who clearly get exposed to these bacilli never come down with the disease. Factors other than exposure also contribute to the likelihood of clinical disease. Host immunity, the amount or duration of exposure, the potency of the bacilli are all factors that could influence whether the disease develops. To make things even more complicated, sometimes the tuberculosis symptoms don't develop until years after the first exposure. So, while the tuberculosis bacilli are a prerequisite for the disease, one cannot say that they alone explain why the disease manifests.

In a similar fashion, while exposure to opioids is a prerequisite to developing the disease of opioid use disorder, and estimates show that 80% of heroin abusers start with prescription painkillers, the vast majority of people who are exposed never come down with the disease.

Opidemic—A Public Health Epidemic

A common estimate is less than 4% of patients prescribed opiates for an acute condition develop the disease. Even among those who abuse heroin, it is not everyone who develops the disease. As stated before, according to current evidence, only about 20% of Vietnam veterans who used heroin ever developed the disease. So, even the use of the potent and illicit opiate, heroin, abused in a stressful context, associated with trauma and the frequent use of all kinds of other addictive substances, we saw the disease spawned in approximately 20% of those exposed. Nonetheless, we commonly assume that heroin is highly addictive and if used it will surely cause an opiate use disorder. What about the 80% who never develop the disease after use of heroin?

Causation from a clinical and scientific standpoint means there must be adequate evidence to reject the null hypothesis. The null hypothesis generally states that no difference occurs between the two groups studied. Causation implies a true difference between the groups studied, and the difference is not able to be explained by potential confounding variables or chance alone. The commonly accepted chance for chance is not 100% but only 95%. Indeed, causation is a complex subject and tied to a solid appreciation of probabilities and statistical understandings. In addition, for formal medical causation to be readily accepted, a plausible explanation as to the mechanism for the result is customarily required. This discussion of causation is often poorly appreciated by most physicians, let alone politicians and the general public.

Bottomline and to avoid the jargon, just because one associates something with something else doesn't mean something caused the other. So while using heroin is highly associated with opioid use disorders, it doesn't mean that use of heroin necessarily causes an opioid use disorder. Clearly, other factors help determine the likelihood for the disease of addiction to occur.

Myth #3—The Drug Causes the Addiction

We have to be careful about blaming a particular substance or drug, or its inherent addictiveness, as the primary cause of a complex phenomenon. Exposure to a substance is understandably a risk factor for a complication from the substance. However, outside of the pharmacology of a substance, other significant risk factors are commonly at play, and these risk factors are oftentimes contextually determined. For example, cholesterol doesn't cause heart disease in most people. Indeed, cholesterol is necessary for life itself! High cholesterol is a risk factor and may contribute to heart disease for those so predisposed.

The same is true with exposure to opioids. Opioids can save lives. It appears though that about 20% of the population is at risk for developing an opioid use disorder or significantly abusing them. Similar to cholesterol, it's not opioids alone which cause the disease. Host factors, how it is used, duration, brain health, social factors, and more all influence the likelihood of abuse and the disease developing.

Opidemic—A Public Health Epidemic

Methadone, a potent and potentially dangerous opioid, is an FDA approved medication to effectively treat patients with opioid uses disorders. It is also inexpensive and highly effective for patients with serious chronic pain disorders. Methadone is an effective treatment largely because it creates stability in the central nervous system, significantly better than shorter acting substances such as morphine or oxycodone. It promotes stability so well that it helps those seriously addicted to opiates function normally! Still, most people and even licensed professionals can't believe or accept that an addictive substance can help someone with an addiction. Methadone is commonly maligned. This is despite evidence so strong that it forced our government to establish methadone clinics.

When attempting to explain the causes of the Opidemic, we are dealing with highly complex biological and social phenomenon. With the complexity, we often seek simple explanations of causation. This happens even among professionals who are well educated and "should know better." In response to the Opidemic, Washington State officials attributed the cause to certain drugs or doses of drugs. The government has fostered billions of dollars in research on finding safer forms of pain pills with a belief that the "abusable" pills prescribed are a significant, if not primary reason, for the Opidemic.

Myth #4—Abstinence Is the Only Answer

Many people still believe that the only true cure from an addiction can come through an abstinence-based approach. Indeed, this belief in abstinence as "the cure" is so strongly held in our country that most formal evaluations for addiction care base their outcomes primarily on the rate of abstinence. It is as if diabetic care was primarily judged by the number of people who were able to abstain from insulin.

Granted, for alcohol use disorders and most substance use disorders, abstinence is a practical and effective surrogate marker for a healthy outcome. However, abstinence is not a universally valid surrogate marker for a healthy outcome with substance use disorders. For example, in moderate to severe opioid use disorders, abstinence is generally contraindicated. Based on the essential need for agonist therapy, the U.S. government, despite all the cultural taboos and myths, has allowed and subsidized methadone clinics.

Myth #5—Bad Doctors

Another variant of blaming the messenger is the common myth that when patients die from an overdose, it means their doctor did something unprofessional. Overdose deaths can be prevented through better support and structure provided by properly educated professionals. There is no doubt about this. Nonetheless, blaming doctors for overdose deaths is similar to blaming a physician for being unprofessional because a percentage of their patients with cancer or heart failure die. In the current climate of bigotry toward physicians who prescribe opioids for pain and sometimes at higher doses than usual, physicians can lose their licenses or DEA registrations, while never being convicted of malpractice![11]

Unsafe prescribing practices in concert with poor diagnostic acumen have undoubtedly contributed to opioid abuse.[12] There are some bad apples and incompetent physicians. Thankfully, these physicians are relatively rare. As in the general population, some physicians are affected by poorly recognized and cared for substance use disorders and mental illnesses. Fortunately, we have longstanding ways to identify and intervene when physicians are incompetent or significantly unprofessional. Even though the occasional doctor will be judged as malpracticing, it is not rational to judge doctors or their prescribing practices as the primary cause of the Opidemic. Hopefully, the reader can appreciate it is a complex subject with multiple risk factors involved.

Opioid use disorders are serious and life-threatening diseases. The suicide rate alone is high. Indeed, some experts estimate that over a

---

[11] Libby RT, *The Criminalization of Medicine - America's War on Doctors*, Praeger Series on Contemporary Health and Living, Westport, Connecticut, 2008 210pgs.

Also visit www.doctorsofcourage.org for a further review and examples of doctors who have been victims of the "War on Drugs."

[12] A full exploration of this is explored in the published paper: An Informal Review of Opioid Dependence (Addiction) Associated with Chronic Opioid Analgesic Therapy (COAT) for Chronic Pain

quarter of the opioid overdoses are forms of suicide. The suicide rate for chronic pain patients is also quite high. Untreated co-occurring disorders are often not recognized or treated in chronic pain patients. Depression, sleep disturbances, other mental conditions, and unrecognized substance use disorders are common in chronic pain patients. All these factors add to the risk for suicide in chronic pain patients.

A common belief remains that physicians and drug companies are to blame for the current epidemic. Authorities quote findings that 80% of heroin users start with prescribed painkillers. The assumption is that the cause of heroin abuse is primarily related to over prescribing by physicians and overzealous marketing by drug companies. While safer and effective options for pain management need to be encouraged, the assumption that stopping the over-prescribing of opioids will eliminate the vast majority of heroin abuse is a myth. While 80% of today's heroin users started by using painkillers, this does not mean that painkillers caused the Opidemic. A more plausible explanation, consistent with the facts, is that the higher availability and access to opioids in susceptible groups generated more people abusing opioids. Indeed, the overdose rate has always been relatively low in the overall subgroup of patients who were prescribed opioids for pain. In certain high risk groups, such as youths or patients on Medicaid, the overdose rates became alarmingly high. Please go back to the discussion above on association versus causation to better appreciate how challenging it can be to determine cause. It is much simpler to determine risk factors. For example, high cholesterol is a risk factor for developing heart disease, but it doesn't cause it. Many people with higher cholesterol levels never suffer from heart disease; and if one lowers one's cholesterol, one may reduce the risk of heart disease, but one doesn't eliminate the possibility.

If one were to conclude that, since the vast majority of motor vehicle accidents occur on city streets, the solution is to simply eliminate as much as possible city streets or vehicles, one would hopefully pause and question the wisdom of such a draconian response. But our strategies with opioid abuse resemble the above example. We proceed as if the only way to curtail MVAs on city streets is to eliminate some city streets (particularly the ones with more accidents!) and proceed with regulatory and even sometimes criminal proceedings against licensed drivers, car dealers, and car manufacturers who contribute to the deaths.

This sort of approach would surely curtail the number of cars on the roads, and as a result there could well be less MVA accidents, at least on the city streets regulated. Imagine, though, the possible unintended consequences of this approach. The financial and social implications are huge. In envisioning this sort of MVA reduction strategy, one can envision some benefits, but the overall strategy is obviously flawed. This comparison is intended to help convey the unsound nature of our current strategies for deterring opioid abuse.

Myth #6—Addicts Are Bad People

Another myth is that addicts are bad or evil, which is their primary problem, and as a result of their behavior they deserve to be locked up or punished. I consider a sociopath the "bad" person. Sociopaths seem incapable of remorse over hurting others. They may be incapable of recognizing socially acceptable behavior and being honest with themselves or others. I do not know what percentage of patients who suffer from opioid use disorders are sociopaths. I have recognized only the rare sociopath in my specialized addiction practice. I conclude that the percentage of sociopaths in relation to those with substance abuse disorders is no greater than in the general population.

There is the old joke about an addict: "How do you know when an addict is lying? Answer: "when they open their mouths!" Most people consider lying a "bad" behavior and this translates into thinking of a liar as a "bad" person. Based on good evidence concerning how many times each day the average person lies, a lot of "bad" people exist out there. Patients in general are known to be dishonest. Diabetic patients and hypertensives are routinely non-adherent and lie to healthcare professionals. In patients with substance use disorders, it is understandable that they would lie. If honest they could suffer significantly and potentially die! People with addictions are not stupid! They have learned that if they tell the truth, they will be highly discriminated against and commonly shamed. Furthermore, with their prescribers, if they are caught or are honest, they could be discharged from ongoing care—and often all care. They are told they must go elsewhere, often without a formal referral.

Opidemic—A Public Health Epidemic

It is expected that when people are stressed, in a state of withdrawal, frustrated or understandably enraged their behavior would be unruly. In addition, it is predictable and natural that patients with a serious substance use disorder are likely to lie or otherwise behave poorly at times secondary to some of the following commonly encountered situations: poorly managed comorbid mental health problems, lack of sleep, acute or chronic pain, lack of money, shortage of trustworthy friends, abuse, frequent reminders that they are "no good and will never amount to anything" or that they are just "low down addicts" who need to be discharged.

No one likes to deal with a liar. We do not feel safe when we cannot trust those with whom we have a relationship. Nonetheless, it is time we start to forgive the lies and get into the solutions. This is the best strategy to put a stop to the lying. Shaming and blaming, if it worked, would have surely resolved the problem by now. In 12-step literature, it is acknowledged that some unfortunates will be incapable of being rigorously honest. This unfortunate character defect is also present far beyond the halls of addiction.

Along the lines of discrimination, when a patient who has an opioid use disorder has chronic pain issues and is not able to adhere to a pain management agreement, they are commonly discharged and not seen for anything anymore. Imagine the level of lying among insulin dependent diabetics, or the rate of adulterated urines one would see, if an insulin dependent diabetic was concerned about being discharged and not prescribed insulin whenever their sugar levels were inordinately high or sugar was ever found in their urine! Medical providers often stigmatize those with addiction for lying. It is known that diabetics or hypertensives are commonly dishonest with their providers. Nonetheless, they rarely suffer as much for lying as an untreated opioid use disorder patient, particularly one who has significant comorbid pain.

A corollary to the myth of people with addictions being bad is the judgement that people with addictions are stupid! The irony is that individuals have the disease, and are still alive, at least in part because they learn so well and have such a hard time forgetting! Those with substance use disorders often have an uncanny ability to cope, read people, make a deal, and put on a performance that surpasses the best of actors. MENSA patients are often the most difficult to treat, in part because they are so smart.

Sadly, and for a variety of reasons, patients with end-stage substance use disorders have damaged their brains, sometimes permanently. One benefit of opioid use disorders compared to some other substance use disorders is that patients, once stabilized, predictably recover normal brain function.

Chapter 3—Substance Abuse: A Public Health Concern

a.) Background

In addition to illicit drug and alcohol abuse, prescription drug abuse is a challenging drug-related problem. In the State of Washington, opioid overdoses related to prescription opiates surpassed motor vehicle accidents as a leading cause of accidental deaths. Mortality and deaths are only part of the grim picture. Health-related issues pertaining to prescription drug abuse and related opioid abuse have broad public health consequences.

When epidemics occur in conjunction with an infectious disease, we are all quite familiar with public health involvement. Effective ways to identify and to limit the spread of a disease are determined and implemented through the expertise of public health officials. The knowledge about the specific agent and the epidemiology of the related disease is coupled with solid public health principles The result is a comprehensive plan for an effective response. Vectors for the disease are reduced, while prompt and effective medical management for the disease is sought. Risk factors for the spread of the disease are identified and are eliminated whenever possible and pragmatic.

An approach similar to the standard public health approach to infectious disease epidemics is needed for our drug abuse epidemic. Public health professionals are trained to discover what works and what doesn't work when considering epidemics. They have training and experience to better assure that a coordination of efforts is made to guarantee the best public health outcomes.

b.) What Has Been Our Approach?

As we have discussed, in our culture we still largely consider opioid abuse as a moral or criminal issue, or at the very least a character flaw in which one is not able to appropriately contend with the myriad of potential stressors of daily life. In contrast, the consensus among well-informed experts is that opioid dependence is a *disease*. The implications are straightforward: attempts to "Just say no" or to eradicate the disease through stiffer penalties, shaming, or other means commonly currently employed are quite likely to fail.

Take for example the HIV epidemic: if we addressed the HIV epidemic with stiffer penalties and simple suggestions such as "Just say no," what would have been the outcome? Even today, at this late date in the HIV epidemic, some would continue to advocate such behavioral approaches. Nonetheless, based on current evidence, the prohibition approach rarely works, particularly when dealing with biological phenomenon. Indeed, the unintended consequences of the "Just say no" approach could easily have aggravated the HIV epidemic. Thankfully, a robust public health response was used to address the HIV epidemic: education was initiated, vectors for the disease were identified, prevention strategies were implemented, and effective treatments initiated. The results demonstrate that this approach is highly successful as compared to prohibition models. While we still have far too many cases of HIV infected people, the incidence and prevalence of the disease have been dramatically reduced, and we have witnessed a relatively dramatic success story through our broad public health approach.

c.) *Explanations for the Lack of a Public Health Response*

The first explanation for the lack of a public health response to substance abuse is one that was already alluded to in the above commentary. A constellation of cultural attitudes and conditioning purports to explain addictive disorders as based on character flaws or even on sinful tendencies. We continue to deny that addictive disorders involving substances are *disease* processes. For this brief discussion, there will be no formal attempt to argue the current scientific evidence that supports substance use disorders, particularly opioid use disorder, as a true disease. Those who still believe that these addictive disorders are not a disease may be asked for a definition of disease. When one uses standard medical means of defining a disease, it quickly becomes evident that most serious substance use disorders are diseases. Opioid use disorders are defined by acknowledged experts as chronic relapsing diseases which, if not properly treated, have a poor prognosis. If the disease concept could be more fully acknowledged, it follows that a public health response to the Opidemic would be more likely.

A second explanation is related to the first. Current institutional and financial systems have left the public health perspective out of the equation. The criminal justice system, social services, and current behavioral addiction services remain the primary players in addressing addictive disorders. While we thankfully have the National Institute for Drug Abuse, the funding for the Centers for Disease Control(CDC), our primary public health agency, is shamefully lacking when it comes to addressing substance abuse problems. If addiction is a disease—and it is arguably our primary public health concern—we must support funding for the CDC and other public health institutions to better prevent and treat substance abuse. Most money funneled to the states through SAMHSA, the federal agency overseeing substance abuse and mental health, go to state services which manage Medicaid and other social services. Unfortunately, they are not directed to public health.

There is a huge "industry" involving suppliers, the criminal justice system, and treatment providers. Based on significant financial incentives, this industry is highly invested in current "markets" and perspectives. It is not that our serious problems stem primarily from corrupt, greedy, or even stupid people. While "profitable" for those offering the service, the case for integrating drug addiction treatment within the criminal justice system is compelling. If someone is arrested for selling opioids or possessing opioids, there is a high chance they have an opioid use disorder. Drug courts have helped assure that some with substance use disorders obtain the care needed to avoid relapses and recidivism. It remains true, however, that current funding and financial incentives compromise not only effective drug court outcomes but also care for those incarcerated. Grievously, an effective public health response has even less funding. We must entertain prevention and early interventions to avoid problems escalating to the point of our criminal justice system becoming involved.

Another possibly important factor in explaining the lack of an effective response to the epidemic is the predilection for objective data. Substance use disorders do not have valid and reliable biomarkers. In contrast, if someone has tuberculosis, we can culture the bacteria. Unfortunately, at least for the time being, comparable biomarkers are not available for substance use disorders. We must depend on reliable and valid clinical tools and expertise.

Another possible explanation for the lack of a robust public health response is that the public wants simple explanations and simple solutions. This goes along with a pattern in our culture to simply blame *someone* or s*omething* as the problem. Recent media coverage of prescription abuse problems in Washington State resulted in many objects of blame: methadone, Medicaid, incompetent physicians, and "drug seekers" were blamed. The state's legislature subsequently passed a law that limited, without a specialist consultation, the ability for most prescribers to prescribe higher doses of opioids.

This new prescription pain medication law is like the political response attempted less than 100 years ago in the way of alcohol prohibition. To address alcohol abuse and its serious public health consequences, prohibition was enacted. It is widely acknowledged that our attempt to prohibit alcohol use was ineffective and likely created more problems than it resolved. The prohibition response appears, however, to remain quite attractive to many Americans. It identifies a complex problem such as alcohol abuse, and then it attempts to simply resolve the problem through a simple solution; that is, to simply create laws to prohibit or limit its use.

While simple explanations and simple solutions often have merit, they have a particularly powerful influence over the electorate. Americans have a peculiar inclination to believe more laws and regulatory efforts will solve all our problems. How else might one explain the ever-burgeoning administrative law in this country? Even when compelling evidence refutes the overall benefit, the electorate is satisfied when their politicians invoke more regulations. Indeed, the regulatory apparatus is arguably the largest financial enterprise in the United States.

In summary, the "Just say no" slogan is a classic example of a simple solution which was politically expedient. When it comes to addressing addictions and the American propensity for addictive disorders, simple explanations and simple solutions have not worked. We need a comprehensive system approach to an inherently complex set of circumstances. A robust public health intervention which incorporates comprehensive system as well as individual interventions is needed.

d.) Issues Specific to Opioids and Opioid Dependence

While there are likely other possible explanations for why the public health perspective appears relatively absent regarding SUDs in general, some issues remain specific to opioids. In relation to opioid abuse, it is especially apparent that a zero-tolerance approach is simply not going to work. Opioids are likely to remain a mainstay of effective and necessary medical care for the foreseeable future. If physicians are not able to prescribe opioids, patients will unnecessarily die and suffer. If opioids are to be prescribed and used effectively, there will be a subgroup of patients who do poorly with them, misuse them, and even die as a result from their use. To some extent, addictive drugs will always be diverted for recreational use. We must not continue to deny the possibility of complications from any effective and potent medical therapy, whether surgical or medical. Statistically, hospitals are dangerous environments!

A reasonable goal is to minimize complications and to ensure that patients who benefit from the medications have reliable access to them. Ongoing medical therapy is commonly essential for opioid use disorders, particularly when patients suffer from comorbid complex pain conditions, other SUDs, or other mental health disorders. Abstinence for most substance use disorders is a good surrogate marker for a solid recovery. However, in the case of moderate to severe opioid use disorders, Medication Assisted Treatment (MAT) is required.

e.) The Answer?

The public health approach uses the best available scientific research to demonstrate what works and what does not work to effectively address an epidemic or public health concern. When needed, further research is encouraged by public health officials. Based on information available, public health professionals coordinate and implement the programs, institutions, and professionals required to effectively address and hopefully resolve the threats. *Effectively* addressing substance abuse problems is well known to have immense cost savings for our government along with the many communities, individuals, and families who deal directly with them.

Pragmatic approaches to solutions are the best, particularly when it comes to challenges that are complex and multifactorial. When attempts to control are demonstrably ineffective and seemingly counterproductive, policies and regulations need to be reevaluated and changed. It is through the collaborative public health model that education regarding problems and solutions can be adequately disseminated on a mass scale—through effectual widespread and local campaigns that promote awareness and access to care in the same vein as they address other epidemics, vaccinations and sexually transmitted diseases. The Federal government works in conjunction with state and local municipalities to connect both urban and rural areas with the same unified agenda. By adopting a public health intervention, attitudes will begin to shift, and new attitudes would not only educate but legitimize and neutralize the issue. Effectively offering treatment on a mass scale would shift a person with a substance use disorder from being considered by society, loved ones or even themselves as a "criminal" or "bad" person who makes "bad" choices to being a patient battling with a long-term disease and worthy of care.

Assuring Proper Medical Care

First, the assurance of proper medical care for those with substance use disorders is needed. The World Health Organization has listed both methadone and buprenorphine as essential medications. Access to both are still quite limited. Opioid use disorders are to be better prevented and better recognized, particularly early on. As already confirmed, the indications for effective agonist therapy (eg: methadone, buprenorphine, etc.) is essential for curbing the epidemic (see Chapter 5 on agonist therapy). A key epidemiological principle states that, in the case of a disease causing an epidemic, to curb the effects of an epidemic it is most often essential to assure effective and timely treatment for the disease. People with opioid use disorders are potential "vectors" for "infecting" other people, and they help maintain a demand for illicit distribution of opioids. Effective care of addictions has been repeatedly demonstrated to limit deaths and unnecessary suffering. While changes in our cultural attitudes, laws, and approaches will curb the Opidemic, we must also provide necessary medical and behavioral care for those with the disease.

Addressing Codependency

"We admitted we were powerless over alcohol—that our lives had become unmanageable."

The above phrase is the first step of Alcoholics Anonymous (AA). Similarly, the first step in Alanon, the fellowship for friends or family of alcoholics, expresses a powerlessness over the behavior of one suffering from alcohol. The focus shifts onto how one can respond differently. The importance of addressing elements of codependence is noteworthy in the discussion of a public health intervention. The process represents an acceptance of a loving detachment vis-a-vis one's own behavior and the behavior of others, particularly those who are dealing with addictive disorders. Paradoxically, this detachment not only helps family and friends but also creates a context in which the person who suffers from an addiction is more likely to improve. When family members or loved ones step away from codependency, the improvement in outcomes from substance use disorders might be as high as 20% or more.

Over time and through working the other steps, the first step of Alanon often translates into an awareness of powerlessness over people, places, and things. This occurs in addition to the acknowledged powerlessness over alcohol or other substances as stated in the first step. The fruition of working the steps can be partially encapsulated into the benefits which rise as a result of saying the serenity prayer:

Opidemic—A Public Health Epidemic

God grant me the serenity to accept the things I cannot change, courage to change the things I can, and the wisdom to know the difference.

We tend to shun from paradoxes. This is true whether they are provided in the form of "The Beatitudes" or as above in the first step of 12-step programs. How does more control come from accepting that we do not have control? If healing is to occur, this is a paradox that the American culture needs to better embrace.

Addressing Misbeliefs and Misunderstandings

No one answer exists to address the amount of misbeliefs and misunderstandings prevalent in our culture as well as in the medical community. A comprehensive approach is needed. The serenity prayer can offer guidance, particularly when dealing with a codependent culture so deeply entrenched in addiction. Let us be willing to question our beliefs. The myths and ignorance surrounding addictions are enormous even among professionals. With the HIV epidemic, public health had to battle enormous misbeliefs and misunderstandings as well as overt stigma in having the infection. I am confident public health could be similarly effective in addressing the Opidemic.

Fewer laws and rules and criminal justice involvement will help, particularly in conjunction with a robust public health and harm reduction approach. I suggest we embrace the best of our Christian heritage: caring for the sick, showing compassion, withholding judgements, and above all being prepared to forgive.

f.) Planning for Our Future

Given the expected delays in implementing a vigorous public health response, let us meanwhile not make things worse in attempts to make things better. The experiments here in Washington to legislate proper medical care for patients with pain have arguably added to the problems associated with beneficial use of opioids and their misuse. In Washington State, while prescription drug-related overdoses have declined, a related increase in heroin overdoses has ensued. Heroin overdoses have proportionally always been the largest public health issue.

It is obvious that less access and less use of opioids are associated with less overdoses and other complications. Quality of life issues and the costs of depriving care also need to be part of comprehensive planning. When people cannot obtain adequate and necessary care legally, they often seek other means. Patients who have opioid use disorders or have serious pain will often seek illicit means of care. If these people don't get care, the evidence is clear they deteriorate and die sooner, and a large number will attempt or succeed at suicide. These are the established facts.

Indeed, as already noted several times, in Northwest Washington surges in heroin use and suicides have occurred following the legislative changes and their implementation. It makes common sense that, if opioids are being used *without proper supervision,* the likelihood of serious complication increase.

Other clinical factors as well may have contributed to the problem of prescription opiate abuse. A critical part of the problem is a gross failure to promptly make the diagnosis of opioid dependence or abuse when it is present. Between 10 and 25% of patients on Chronic Opioid Analgesic Therapy meet the criteria for opiate use disorder. Another important factor is our negligence in effectively and adequately treating the disease when it is identified, and perhaps most importantly it is our gross failure to recognize the risk factors for the development of the disease and to initiate proper preventive measures. Similar conditions, if not effectively recognized, would fuel the spread of any disease and epidemic.

Third parties, particularly the Medicaid system, which has a high percentage of addicted and high-risk patients, poorly reimburses physicians and other suitable clinicians for formal screening and treatment of drug abuse problems. In the past they have even harassed such providers based on the false premise that these patients only require behavioral care. Effective medical and behavioral treatment needs to be readily available for those with the disease. Similarly, if proper screening and prevention efforts were taken, as with cancer, the development or progression of the disease would be curtailed. As already stated, the cost savings would be enormous.

While progress is obvious, in Washington State we still have systems and policies in place that serve to minimize the importance of medical care for addiction. While behavioral care is available, it is the criminal justice system that "feeds" and maintains it. We continue to see the criminal justice system (the hammer) as the main access to "treatment."

As already noted, we tend to blame prescribing clinicians, patients, drug companies, and even the drugs themselves. While these simple explanations have political appeal, we need effective solutions that remove the simple and appealing blame games. In review of evidence and extensive clinical experience, when it comes to dealing effectively with addictions, no evidence purports that blaming offers any worthwhile results, particularly in the long run.

We must entertain system solutions (ie: a public health perspective) rather than to blame one another or to find scapegoats. We are always going to have incompetent or corrupt professionals, sociopaths, and criminals as well as good and bright people addicted to substances. An ability and capacity to effectively address these impaired members of our community is called for. Arguably, the need is greater than monitoring cholesterol or even sugar levels. It is our young who are especially succumbing to the disease.

Regulatory agencies often go too far and have been provided too much authority. All the evidence and clinical experience supports specialized medical care is part of the solution rather than part of the problem. Qualified and capable physicians have nonetheless experienced the full weight of regulatory enforcement. This has been touched upon repeatedly, and the book "Criminalization of Medicine—America's War on Doctors" by Ronald T. Libby documented the pattern even back in

2008. When regulatory agents cannot readily distinguish friend from foe, as has been frequently the case, one must assume the presence of a significant system problem.

Europe has made significant progress to decriminalize substance abuse and make the use of substances a public health problem rather than a criminal one. Portugal has led the way. Switzerland and other European countries are following with consistently impressive results. Perhaps we can learn from others' experiences and mitigate our propensity to think our way is the best? The Chinese and other dictatorial regimes have even tried the death penalty for drug dealers. Has that worked? The answer is no and at what cost? Most of the illicit fentanyl and other substances on our streets often comes from China.

In summary, our system problems related to substance abuse and misuse cry out for a radical change. Let us take resources from the regulatory sphere and move them preferably to the public health realm. Public health respects and promotes system changes. While system changes are not simple or straightforward, they are often needed in order to effectively and durably confront a public health crisis.

The following chapter explores more background components of the public health perspective. I examine epidemiology, the study of epidemics. In the next chapter, agonist therapy and medication assisted treatment (MAT) are reviewed. In the last chapter, I review the medical uses of substances that are addictive. Based on our expected ongoing use of addictive substances and the nature of our brains, we are not going to eliminate substance use disorders. Our objective must be a public health response in which harm reduction and effective prevention strategies dominate.

Chapter 4—Epidemics and Epidemiology

a.) Definition of an Epidemic

Epidemics[13] are commonly associated with outbreaks of infectious diseases: flu, polio, tuberculosis, swine flu, AIDS, Zika virus, food-related pathogens, and many others. An epidemic may reflect the presence of any disease or health-threatening process that occurs out of the ordinary. In public health circles, epidemics reflect higher than normal morbidity (disabilities) and mortality (deaths) in groups of people (populations).

b.) What Epidemiologists Do

Epidemiologists track levels of morbidity and mortality; they alert the public to changes in trends. Once an epidemic is identified, they are trained to identify likely causes and promote effective remedies. Public health professionals are familiar with the science of epidemiology—the science which promotes the understanding of and effective responses to epidemics.

---

[13] Merriam Webster's Definition of Epidemic.

Epidemiology is a science which depends highly on statistics. Statistics reflect data compiled through conventional forms of mathematics and permit informed professionals to predict trends, causes, and effective responses. The average person associates a truth with what can be expected with near certainty. For example, water freezing at 32'F or 0'C is a truth commonly accepted by most people. In the realm of living systems, this level of certainty is rarely encountered. To improve their ability to predict, epidemiologists do not base their predictions on specific, individual experiences; they are trained to base them on the experience of large groups of people. It is the study of groups or populations which allows an epidemiologist to provide a statistical probability for predicting risks for and effective responses to an epidemic.

While most people do not understand nuclear physics, they do accept what a nuclear bomb can do. Similarly, while epidemiology is not well understood by the average person, epidemiology does save lives and sometimes in dramatic ways. The epidemiologist is for populations what the physician is for the individual. Epidemiologists help us place good bets regarding our collective health, similar to the way a physician places good bets for the health of a patient.[14]

---

[14] Rotchford JK, *Letting the Horses Run, Patient Care*, 1998, October 30, pp.123-24.

c.) Do Statistics Lie?

Based on the outright abuse which can come from poorly interpreted and inappropriately applied statistics, people often believe that statistics lie and that no real truth can be gained in statistics. As with most facts, statistical facts are commonly interpreted through the lens of beliefs. Any good politician, let alone salesman, and even some professionals may misuse statistics in a way to support their ends. This does not mean that statistics lie. It does infer, though, that statistics are commonly misinterpreted and misused. Most often the misinterpretation comes from ignorance as well as through the clouded lens of our beliefs.

In contrast, a good epidemiologist can be delighted when a long held belief is questioned. For an epidemiologist, beliefs are supposed to be questioned. Beliefs are to be changed on evidence, evidence that can be independently evaluated and found to be highly predictive of what is likely to happen. Furthermore, a good epidemiologist will more likely speak in probabilities rather than certainties. The relative certainties of some aspects of the physical world are not to be expected in living systems, where probabilities are the rule rather than the exception.[15]

---

[15] The Five Most Popular Ways Statistics Lie – Link to an outside source for review.

Lies, Damn Lies, and Statistics – Link to the Wikipedia discussion of the topic.

d.) The Interplay Between Facts and Beliefs

As a physician with a solid background in epidemiology, for a long time I believed that facts and objective realities dominate what happens in our lives. I no longer believe this. When it comes to understanding human responses and how best to predict them, I now believe one must emphasize beliefs, conditioning, and contextual variables as being more relevant than the facts.

Our beliefs are more likely to influence the facts, rather than facts influencing our beliefs. The proverbial "I'll believe it when I see it" becomes "I will see it when I believe it." Despite a shift in my beliefs, gained over a lifetime of medical practice, I do not abandon the importance of facts. Facts can be used to alter beliefs—at least I hope so. Furthermore, I believe that facts (objective evidence) support my belief that one's interpretation of facts is commonly trumped by beliefs. When it comes to remembering facts, one's beliefs, conditioning and expectations are especially important to predict how facts will be interpreted. Commonly, based on the objective filming of an event, eye witnesses—who testify under oath to have vividly remembered seeing the facts—can be shown to have grossly misinterpreted them.

In addition to the facts and educational background, other variables predict human behavior. For example, about 80% of the population, when demanded to do so by an authoritative figure, will routinely behave significantly outside of, and even contrary to their established values and norms of predicted behavior.

e.) Complex Causes of Epidemics and Practical Implications

The previous discussion of the role of beliefs in interpreting facts is particularly relevant when we discuss the cause of an epidemic. The cause for an epidemic, despite the science involved, is steeped in cultural as well as individual beliefs. Perhaps the best argument I can make for this is to provide examples of where the purported or accepted cause for a medical condition, let alone an epidemic, is based primarily on cultural and other conditioned beliefs rather than objective evidence.

Take the simple example of a physician reporting to their patient a cause for their medical findings. A common example may be a case of appendicitis. This is a relatively common treated medical condition. The facts support an inflamed intestinal appendage as the cause which, when left untreated, can burst and be fatal. The pathologist's objective report confirms the diagnosis based on objective findings common to other patients with signs and symptoms of appendicitis. Despite the obvious pragmatic value in this belief system, let me formally question its ultimate truth. It is a fact that some patients with signs and symptoms of appendicitis get better despite not having surgery. Is it because they don't have appendicitis? Or is it because of other variables and truths which may speak to other pathologies and possible solutions? In Chinese medicine, with thousands of years of useful outcomes, the explanation for the signs and symptoms of appendicitis are entirely different from our Western explanations. Like the nature of light itself, which from one perspective behaves like a wave and another like photons, both are "true," while not exclusively so.

Common experience acknowledges that after the appendix is removed, symptoms or complications from appendicitis are unlikely. These facts do not preclude, however, that a patient's distinct nature, their diet, current circumstances, anatomy, and context may better explain the signs and symptoms related to what we commonly label "appendicitis." These other variables might be considered causes similar to the way high blood pressure is commonly considered to cause strokes. More accurately, hypertension dependent on its severity, is a significant risk for having a stroke.

In our culture, in surgical matters such as appendicitis, we attribute the cause to the final and objective pathology findings of appendicitis. In Western medicine, we strongly believe in the value of objective facts and findings. While as previously noted, the pragmatic value of honoring the objective is hard to deny, the importance one puts on the objective is subjective; and eventually it filters down to subjective beliefs and values of right or wrong, healthy or unhealthy, beautiful or ugly, and other polarities. A public health official may believe that reducing overall morbidity and mortality (measurable entities) is the most important outcome. A politician, a military leader, or a religious leader may believe otherwise.

Another example in clinical medicine is when clinicians use the diagnosis of depression as the cause of a sign or symptom. As with many Western diagnoses and labels, causes are often discussed in the context of the solutions provided. For example, if a person has signs and symptoms of depression and gets better with a prescription for an antidepressant, it is commonly assumed that the cause for the patient's signs and symptoms was depression. This is not acceptable reasoning and represents a form of the *post hoc ergo propter hoc* fallacy: "After this, therefore because of this." As discussed already in Chapter 2, this fallacy commonly occurs even among professionals; it remains widespread in clinical medicine as well as in other disciplines exploring and explaining causes.

Multiple examples exist in which the illusion of simple explanations for cause and effect are applied to complex events. When it comes to human behavior, whether in the realms of economics, politics, religion, let alone medicine and public health, humility is indicated. Simple explanations of causes are better regarded in terms of appreciating risks and probabilities. Rather than explain a heart attack based on a blood vessel clotting, as true as it might be, it is important to consider other potential impacts—genetics, diet, exercise, obesity, non-specific cultural factors, anger, stress, inflammation, hypertension, hyperlipidemia, diabetes, age, Monday mornings, hormonal abnormalities—to our understandings of "the cause."

Opidemic—A Public Health Epidemic

With the above discussion in mind, simple explanations for complex phenomenon are commonly problematic. The attempt to seek simple answers has been evident in how we commonly try to explain the opioid epidemic, let alone any epidemic. Is heroin the cause of our opioid epidemic? Is it oxycodone? Is it now fentanyl? Is it related to high doses of medications? Is it Big Pharma? Is it the prescribing practices of physicians? Is it morally deficient people? Is it people who are not able to "Just say no?" Is it a lack of adequate regulatory efforts? Or might "the cause" simply relate to our human nature and the question of access and probabilities?

Simple explanations often satisfy the general public, the media, or politicians, but most often do not promote comprehensive and effective solutions. In clinical medicine we have learned to appreciate the importance of not assuming the value of an intervention without studying it thoroughly. Perhaps regulators could learn from clinical medicine? For example, similar to the protections we have in place before a new pharmaceutical can come on the market, let's formally test new regulations. With pharmaceuticals, even with clear and established mechanisms of actions (purported causes) in addition to apparent predicted favorable benefit to risk outcomes, extensive controlled trials are required before we allow a new pharmaceutical to be marketed. Furthermore, extensive follow-up and monitoring for long-term, unintended consequences are required. Even with these protections in place—including all our efforts to minimize the effects of beliefs and profit motivations through random selection of samples, blinding of patients and providers, and other rigorous aspects of clinical study, designs and analyses—some FDA approved pharmaceuticals do not measure up to the test of time.

In contrast, governments and politicians exhibit little hesitation to impose significant interventions in the enactment of new laws and regulations. I have already spoken to some of the unintended consequences of regulatory efforts in Washington State and those stemming from DEA involvement. The benefits of such regulatory efforts are problematic, particularly if one looks at them in light of their unintended consequences. Explaining the causes or severity of the opioid abuse epidemic as being entirely, or even significantly attributed to physician prescribing practices, or the doses of medications prescribed is flatly unsubstantiated by the evidence. The evidence that has been provided for these arguments is at best in the realm of associations with a callous disregard for prominent confounding variables. Objectively, we have spent valuable resources with limited benefits in combating substance abuse and misuse. In addition, the unintended consequences from our current approaches are numerous and serious.

f.) Complex Problems and Unintended Consequences

As to the unintended consequences of such regulatory interventions as seen in Washington State, we note that, while overdose deaths associated with prescribed opioids went down, heroin overdoses skyrocketed, and heroin overdoses always represented a major share of overdose deaths.

The gateway theory of prescription opiates being the cause of opioid use disorders has solid credibility. It is impossible to develop the disease, no matter what one's other risk factors are, if one is never exposed repeatedly to opioids! Nonetheless, to ascribe the exposure as being a primary cause is problematic. One can never eradicate exposure to opioids given their fundamental and established role in medicine.

The regulatory efforts have surely limited access to medical care desperately needed by some, many with serious, disabling, or life-threatening conditions. Might the fear of regulatory consequences, losing one's license, and even criminal charges, make it challenging for physicians to justify treating complex pain patients with opioids, let alone providing appropriate care to those with opioid use disorders? The increased shortage and public health crisis stemming from the lack of physicians willing to treat complex pain patients suggests serious unintended consequences of the regulatory efforts aimed at physician prescribing. The significant morbidity and mortality associated with untreated chronic pain are not disputed. Opioids are commonly the only viable option available.

In my published case report, *A Complex Pain Patient Who is Opioid Dependent*, I make a compelling argument for the serious consequences, often unrecognized, when patients with chronic pain and co-occurring opioid use disorders do not receive adequate agonist therapy. Indeed, even the Washington State Pain Rules themselves, based on overwhelming evidence, affirm that the prognosis is poor for patients with moderate to severe opioid use disorders who do not receive appropriate agonist therapy. In another peer reviewed journal, An Informal Review of Opioid Dependence (Addiction) Associated with Chronic Opioid Analgesic Therapy (COAT) for Chronic Pain, convincing evidence suggests that as many as twenty percent of patients on opioids for chronic pain have a significant opioid use disorder. Given the above information, legitimate public health concerns must arise when these chronic pain patients lose access to appropriate opioid therapy.

If one does the math, the pain rules have likely generated substantially more unnecessary deaths, let alone morbidity, than they prevented. Imagine the public outrage if a pharmaceutical agent with even less risks had been allowed to be marketed.

g.) A Public Health Response Is Needed

The above discussion provides warnings against oversimplifying complex phenomenon such as the Opidemic. Dealing with epidemics is best left to professionals who can be relatively insulated from political and cultural biases and beliefs. Our public health officials and the epidemiologists they employ are the trained professionals with the expertise to respond based on the best evidence for positive outcomes. They are trained to analyze and respond to complex problems that threaten our public health. Because substance abuse is just beginning to be recognized as a public health concern, these officials will face a steep learning curve. This is reflected in part by the CDC's recent involvement in publishing recommendations for the use of opioids in pain management.

Chapter 5—Agonist Therapy for Opioid Misuse

a.) Definitions

Agonist therapy[16] is the term associated with the use of medications that stimulate nerve cell receptors (mu receptors and others) in the brain. These medications stimulate receptors similar to the way natural and internal chemicals do. The intent of prescribed agonists in the context of pain management or addiction management is to stabilize and improve brain function.

Opiates or opioids: opiates are substances derived from the poppy plant. The term opioid means any substance that behaves like an opiate. Some medications such as methadone are synthesized and act similar to those substances directly derived from the poppy plant. For practical purposes, whether the substance comes from the actual poppy plant or not, opioids act similarly, and they can all be associated with addiction or opioid use disorders.

Opiate dependence is the past medical diagnosis for patients who are addicted to opioids, ie: have an opioid use disorder. As discussed

---

[16] agonist therapy online definition

previously in Chapter 1, well established (DSM IV) diagnostic criteria determine the diagnosis of opiate dependence. Opioid dependence requires meeting 3 or more of the following criteria occurring during a 12 month period. Recently, DSM 5 criteria for opioid use disorders were developed for mild, moderate, and severe opioid use disorders. These criteria better reflect that like most diseases, particularly chronic ones, the severity and consequences of the disease can vary greatly. Note DSM 5 criteria are not as vetted as the DSM IV criteria, and some experts are not in agreement with DSM 5 eliminating markers of physical dependence in patients being managed with prescription opiates.

(1) Tolerance, as defined by either of the following:

(a) markedly increased amounts of the substance needed to achieve intoxication or desired effect

(b) a markedly diminished effect with continued use of the same amount of the substance

(2) Withdrawal, as manifested by either of the following:

(a) characteristic withdrawal syndrome

(b) the same (or a closely related) substance is taken to relieve or avoid withdrawal symptoms

(3) Larger amounts of the substance is taken over a longer period of time than intended.

(4) A persistent desire or unsuccessful efforts to cut down or control substance use.

(5) A great deal of time is spent obtaining the substance, using the substance or recovering from its effects.

(6) Important social, occupational, or recreational activities are given up or reduced because of substance use.

(7) Substance use is continued despite having a persistent, recurrent physical or psychological problem that is either caused or exacerbated by the substance.

Some arguments may arise over these criteria, particularly in cases of patients who are being prescribed opiates for painful conditions. One may sometimes hear the term "pseudoaddiction" used. The behavior of patients who are not receiving good pain management often mimics the behavior of a patient with an addictive disorder. Indeed, it is frequent to see an overlap between the behavior in chronic pain patients and those with addictive disorders. Furthermore, patients who are addicted often suffer from pain, particularly if they are being prescribed controlled substances. Body pain is also commonly experienced at times of opioid withdrawal. Whether an opioid is properly prescribed and taken or used illegally, its use can induce the disease of an opioid use disorder, particularly in susceptible individuals. Even some grade school children know that oxycodone can be considered weak heroin in a pill form.

As already explained in Chapter 1, some opioids are more likely to promote addiction than others. For example, people who regularly use heroin are more likely to become addicted than people who regularly use codeine. Nonetheless, over periods of time, even weak opiates used by a predisposed patient can and do lead to addiction.

b.) *Role of a Specialized Pain and Addiction Medical Practice*

In a specialized pain management practice, patients are referred because their pain is poorly controlled. If the referred patient has been prescribed opioids over some time, given the above criteria for opioid dependence, it is not uncommon for a diagnosis of opiate use disorder to be justified.[17] Notably, this may even be true when the patient is no longer using opiates! Referred patients are often struggling, and opioids are frequently an issue. They are an issue, whether it is about taking too much or too little. Concerns and preoccupation around a substance is a marker for addiction, and a good percentage of the patients referred for specialized care meet formal criteria of an opioid use disorder.

Patients who currently take or who have taken pain pills, and have done so only as prescribed, may still have an opioid use disorder. While an inability to adhere to medical recommendations brings up red flags, it must be appreciated that when a patient is currently abstinent or not using opioids, this does not exclude the possibility of them having an

---

[17] Rotchford, JK. *Opioids in Chronic Pain Management - A Guide for Patients.* Port Townsend: Olympas Medical Services, 2018, print.

opioid use disorder. The diagnostic criteria apply to any 12 month period in a patient's life, whether it is recent or 20 years or more in the past. Like any substance use disorder, opiate use disorders are chronic and lifetime disorders. Once the brain has been programmed, it cannot readily forget for it has been designed to remember. As in coming to speak a foreign language, over time one can forget much of what one has learned. But if one learned a language as a youth or spoke it for some time, one will probably retain significant amounts of it. The same holds true for the language of addiction.

One can learn other languages and take measures to avoid using the language of addiction, but once learned, it is virtually impossible to entirely forget it, whether one wants to forget it or not. Just as some people learn foreign languages easier than others, likewise, especially if one is relatively young, some are naturally more prone to learn and acquire the language of addiction.

Conversely, for the elderly population it is quite difficult to develop an addiction, particularly if one has never before suffered from any other sort of addiction. How easy is it for a sixty-year-old to learn a foreign language, particularly if they've never learned one before? In general, it is quite difficult if not impossible to learn a foreign language late in life. The same holds true with addiction. For this reason, one is not to be very concerned about a sixty-plus-year-old, who has never had a substance use disorder, developing an opioid use disorder of any significance. This comparison with language acquisition is even clinically helpful in understanding and accepting the realities of preventing and treating addictive disorders.

Furthermore, addiction involves more than withdrawal and tolerance to a substance. Physical dependence, as reflected by signs of withdrawal or tolerance, almost always occurs in patients who take significant amounts of opioids for more than a week or so and can occur as well with the use of non-addicting substances. Substance use disorders (addiction) by medical definition involve much more than physical dependence.

The vast majority of patients with moderate to severe opioid use disorders require ongoing agonist therapy (treatment with long acting opioids) for optimal health. The diagnosis implies that permanent changes to the brain have occurred. As a result, many patients with the disease who do not receive adequate agonist therapy could be described as being in a state of chronic subacute withdrawal, often poorly appreciated even by an astute clinician.

Risk factors exist for opioid use disorders. If someone is relatively young at first use, becomes energized with opiate use, has had other addictions or co-morbid mental disorders, or has experienced abuse or other serious traumas in their life, and has taken opioids regularly (whether prescribed or not) during a 6-12 month period, it is reasonable to treat them as though they have an opioid use disorder. When a patient who was repeatedly exposed to opioids meets several of these risk factors, in my experience they nearly always meet 3 out of the 12 DSM

IV criteria. If a patient is envisioning long-term opioid therapy for a painful condition and has significant risk factors, it is reasonable to treat them as if they have an opioid use disorder. It is of course best to prevent the disease from developing in the first place.

c.) *Treatment of Opioid Use Disorders Under DSM–V Criteria*

Below is a quote from page 10 of Washington State's Interagency Guideline on Opioid Dosing for Chronic Non-cancer Pain, published in March 2007:

Prognosis is poor for patients with a DSM diagnosis of opioid dependence or opioid abuse who do not receive opioid agonist therapy, such as Methadone or Buprenorphine (Sees 2000, Kakko 2003).

Treatment of opiate dependency with the best outcomes includes medical agonist therapy as well as behavioral care. Abstinence-based approaches (no pharmacological support) appear to have long-term favorable outcomes only in a minority of patients (perhaps no more than 1 in 20). However, even in the 5% of cases who maintain an abstinence approach, the question remains: what constitutes optimal outcomes? If one defines "success" of opioid use disorders based simply on abstinence from an opiate, this sidesteps the question of how best to promote optimal health. Most rational people would not judge success simply on the basis of whether a patient is taking or not a medication. *The most important medical outcomes have to do with indicators of quality and duration of life!*

This is why any good physician prescribes any medication. Simply put, good medicine is more likely to promote health than detract from it.

The level of abstinence from alcohol might be a reasonable and sound marker for a favorable outcome for a patient who has an alcohol use disorder. In contrast, total abstinence from opioids clearly has a poor long-term prognosis in patients who have opioid use disorders. Similarly, a good percentage of patients who are addicted to nicotine will actually live longer if they are provided lifetime agonist therapy with nicotine or nicotine-like substances.

With professional medical care, it is essential to do all one can to help patients achieve favorable outcomes regarding whatever disease they are confronting. Optimal health is the outcome sought after for all diseases. Chronic pain and substance use disorders are diseases which cause much suffering and are associated with high morbidity and mortality. While informed professionals do not routinely recommend abstinence-based approaches for opioid use disorders, it is obviously important to take measures for judicious and professionally supervised medication use, and to assure that medicines prescribed are used as prescribed.

An abstinence-based approach in the context of a serious chronic pain disorder or complicating psychiatric disorders is obviously less likely to be associated with good outcomes. While this appears self evident, many medical colleagues and addiction professionals continue to routinely encourage abstinence-based approaches. While the risks of diversion and abuse are present with agonist therapy, with proper care and monitoring the risks are acceptable compared to the documented benefits. The literature supports that access to effective treatment for opioid use disorders reduces problematic opioid use not only for the individual but for our entire community. Both methadone and buprenorphine have been qualified as "essential medicines" by the World Health Organization(WHO).

It is often difficult for a patient with an OUD to make rational choices regarding the use of their medications. This is particularly true early on in recovery. In addition to the lack of insight and judgement associated with addictive disorders, social pressures, laws, conditioning, and taboos often dominate rational decision making both on the part of patients and unfortunately professionals as well. One can believe in a loving God and, with God's grace and a host of other contextual factors, an abstinence-based approach does sometimes work. Nonetheless, given the current medical evidence, in patients who meet formal criteria for a moderate to severe opioid use disorder, an abstinence-based approach must not be recommended, especially to begin with. The comparable benefits of long acting naltrexone is still being debated as an alternative to agonist therapy for opioid use disorders. When chronic pain or other mental disorder co-occur, we can expect naltrexone to have a much more limited role.

Since perceived choice is so highly valued in our culture, services must acknowledge a patient's right to choose an abstinence approach. If an abstinence approach is elected, one must mitigate the consequences of what is professionally considered a "bad bet." This approach is consistent with the Hippocratic Oath. Hence, patients who have an opioid use disorder and are suffering from chronic pain should expect the utmost support from their healthcare team, whether or not a patient's decision is consistent with standards for safe and effective treatment.

Chapter 6—Medical Uses of Addictive Substances

Addictive substances have an essential role in medical care. This is confirmed by extensive research and extensive clinical experience. Addictive substances also have serious side effects. Furthermore, when used inappropriately, addictive substances can be fatal. This brief review is intended to help promote safe and effective uses of addictive substances. As discussed previously, abstinence from potentially addictive substances is not necessarily part of a safe and effective solution. When considering a robust public health response, it is paramount to consider the medically pertinent uses of certain substances. Principles common to all addictive disorders are shared. Next, a limited discussion specific to commonly prescribed addictive substances is provided.

a.) General Principles

Herein, I provide a warranted repetition and, in some cases, an elaboration of principles explored in Chapter 1 under the subject *Basic Understanding of Addiction and Opioid Use Disorders*.

First, I want to reiterate and correct a common misconception: addiction is not synonymous with physical dependence. Many substances associated with physical dependence are not addictive, and some addictive substances cause little or no physical dependence. Physical dependence implies that physiological changes have resulted from the repeated use of a substance. These changes may create symptoms of withdrawal when the substance is stopped or reduced. While with some substances withdrawal is a minor concern, other addictive substances are associated with potentially life-threatening withdrawal. Physical dependence is also associated with tolerance. Tolerance is the term used to describe how, over time, a greater dose of a substance is required for it to have a similar therapeutic or "high" effect.

Addictive substances have one physiological effect in common: all addictive substances cause a pharmacologically induced release of dopamine in an area of the brain described as the reward center. This center is in the front of the brain and its "main processor" is called the nucleus accumbens. Ups and downs of dopamine in the nucleus accumbens are required for addictive patterns to emerge. Indeed, a flux in dopamine levels appears to be the primary determinant of all forms of higher learning. When dopamine levels are maintained stable, as with the use of long-acting opioids such as methadone or buprenorphine, addictive patterns are often arrested and are much less likely to progress.

Addictions are not a function of simply using a substance over time. As the result of using an addictive substance over time cues, triggers, and outside factors are part of what is learned. It is the use of a substance based on a cue or a craving which is an important hallmark of a substance use disorder. Addictions imply dysfunction in areas of the brain which are largely subconscious, such as the activity in the nucleus accumbens. For the most part, addictions involve dysfunction in broad areas of the limbic system. The limbic system helps us manage emotions, relationships, pain, and sleep, among other things. Because addictive substances strongly influence the limbic system, these substances are commonly used to effectively treat dysfunctions and stress in the limbic system. Addictive substances are a "double edged sword" for, while they may help normalize limbic system function, they also can contribute to limbic system dysfunction, particularly when misused or with long-term use.

Short-term use of addictive substances is not commonly associated with the development of addictive patterns. Like most learned behavior, repetition over time is the best predictor of a learned behavior. People are more or less vulnerable to become addicted based on their genetics as well as past experiences. Cultural variables are still being explored as to their degree of risk, but they clearly play an important role.

Addictive disorders are chronic and relapsing disorders, and like most chronic diseases the causes are complex. As already stated, they are associated with genetic as well as environmental variables. A substance use disorder can never be entirely cured, because it involves memory. Human beings have evolved to remember well. Short of developing dementia, most people remember well, even if only on a subconscious level. The "rewards" associated with using an addictive substance are inevitably registered as "important" to a healthy brain. It follows that rather than "forgetting" the patterns of addiction, a better long-term strategy is to learn new patterns of responding to life events.

For example, if one intended to no longer speak English, a good strategy would be immersion in learning and speaking only a foreign language. "Just saying no" to speaking English is unlikely to be the most productive strategy in the long run. The same is true regarding abstinence from addictive substances. Outside input and support is essential for a good prognosis, and repetition of any newly learned pattern is always helpful. As in learning a foreign language, independent study is limited in establishing new behaviors associated with the prevention and responses linked with substance use disorders (SUDs). It works so much better to work and talk with others conversant in the language of recovery!

b.) Issues Pertinent to Opioids

The effective management of opioid use disorders highlights the above principles perhaps better than any other SUD. The epidemic of opioid overdoses has caught public attention. In some states, the death rate has surpassed that of motor vehicle accidents. Even the Center for Disease Control (CDC) is now involved. Pundits are clamoring to limit the prescribing of opiates, and many professionals are advising that patients must be taken off of all chronic opioids unless they are soon to die of cancer. These opinions exist despite overwhelming evidence that opioids in the proper context provide for the best health outcomes, often much better than other current alternatives.

Opidemic—A Public Health Epidemic

Based on the principles of addiction, it is understandable that methadone and buprenorphine (two modern opioids) have efficacy in patients who are addicted to opiates. They are long-acting substances, and when properly prescribed and used (limited self-medicating), there is abundant evidence as to their benefits. They both allow for stable levels of dopamine. Conversely, abstinence approaches with moderate to severe opioid use disorders have poor outcomes. In one formal study in Sweden, the mortality was 20% after one year of treatment that included only behavioral support compared to 5% with agonist therapy (methadone or buprenorphine). Regarding morbidity, the available evidence demonstrates that agonist therapy is much more effective than behavioral therapy alone.

Opioids are quite safe for long-term use compared to many medications used to treat chronic diseases. Patients can readily live long and productive lives when properly using opioids. Some side effects are associated with opioids, and steps to address complications are important. Complications can arise from their abuse, interaction with other substances, hormone disturbances, constipation, and even sleep apnea. Fortunately, appropriate professional oversight can minimize these complications.

The tendency in clinical care is to use the least number of opiates as possible and to get patients off opiates as soon as possible. When opiates are used for short duration (acute illnesses), this approach makes good clinical sense, particularly when safer or as effective alternatives are readily available. With chronic illnesses, however, as in patients with an opioid use disorder, the attachment to having patients entirely off of opioids is dysfunctional. Nonetheless, this attachment is common and is reflected in the research. Current research in opiate use disorders commonly indicate abstinence as an outcome of success. This is quite striking. No other chronic disease has abstinence as a preferred outcome. This is particularly true for abstinence from proven effective medical therapy. Why minimize therapy simply for the sake of minimizing therapy? Better health outcomes consistent with social values are the objective of proper medical care and health related policies.

With most substance use disorders, abstinence is a valuable surrogate marker for healthy long-term outcomes. It makes common sense to not use more of any medicine than is indicated. Nonetheless, in all other areas of medicine, the quality of life (morbidity) and death rates (mortality) are the primary indicators of effective therapy. If a patient can benefit from less insulin or blood pressure medicine because of weight loss, this is beneficial. But we agree on this not simply because the patient is taking less insulin. We consider the weight loss beneficial because the weight loss and need for less medications are associated with better outcomes, not worse ones!

The above peculiarities of how we deal with opioid use disorders is associated with some of the aforementioned cultural issues and the lack of biomarkers to evaluate progress in the treatment of substance use disorders. If there were clear biomarkers that measured stress or other indicators of good health in patients in recovery, similar to the markers we have in managing diabetes or hypertension, the emphasis on getting patients off of all medications would likely be tempered.

Most problems involving chronic central nervous system problems, such as chronic pain and substance use disorders wax and wane significantly over time. All good clinical measures for mental illnesses as well as SUDs must take this into account. Some patients with opioid use disorders who receive proper behavioral care can do quite well for six months or so, while the brain is compensating from the sudden change to abstinence. It is often after some time when relapses occur—and then the consequences can be fatal. The consequences due to ongoing chronic stress from sub-acute withdrawal is also a major concern when evaluating long-term morbidity associated with abstinence-based approaches.

c.) *Issues with Benzodiazepines*

Perhaps no substance use disorder is as challenging to manage as those associated with benzodiazepines: Lorazepam (Ativan), Clonazepam (Klonopin), Diazepam (Valium), Librium (Chlordiazepoxide), etc. Outside of hospitalization or serious long-term behavioral care and gradual tapering, the prognosis is commonly guarded. The withdrawal from benzodiazepines can be life threatening and best done only under professional and ideally specialized care.

As with opiate use disorders, comorbid mental health problems are common with benzodiazepine use disorders and need to be effectively addressed. The combination of opioids and benzodiazepines is especially problematic because of its association with a large number of fatal overdoses. Furthermore, it is commonly pertinent to recognize that patients who continue to take both tend not to improve. This appears to be true whatever the presenting conditions or symptoms are.

Short-term use of benzodiazepines can be very helpful and most appropriate in a number of medical contexts. However, if one has a history of a substance use disorder, self-medicating, the use of benzodiazepines must be closely monitored and ideally tapered over time. Benzodiazepines can be particularly problematic for patients who have abused alcohol. A significant overlap occurs in the receptors affected by both alcohol and benzodiazepines.

d.) Issues with Stimulants

Methamphetamine abuse remains a scourge for many rural communities. Methamphetamine is highly addictive and has been demonstrated to be toxic to the brain with sometimes long-term brain damage. As with cocaine, a social element needs to be appreciated and addressed. It is essential that all patients with SUDs develop a supportive community outside of their fellow abusers. This appears to be especially vital for patients who have methamphetamine use disorders.

When long-acting methylphenidate or amphetamine salts are used to treat ADHD, there appears to be very little evidence of abuse or addictive patterns emerging, even in patients at high risk. Nonetheless, all stimulants, despite dose or delivery, are deemed highly addictive by the FDA & DEA.

e.) Issues with Medical Cannabis[18]

Depending on context and how it is used and taken, the addictive and other side effects from cannabis use are minimal compared to most prescribed addictive medications. Regular cannabis use for medical purposes is particularly safe after the brain has matured, after the age of 25 or so. It is estimated that 15% of the larger population will become addicted to cannabis when using it for recreational purposes. Physical dependence can occur, but is less apparent than with many other addictive substances. Someone older than 60, who has never had an addictive disorder or other significant mental illness, is very unlikely to become addicted to cannabis, even if they smoke it, which is relatively contraindicated for medical purposes.

For medical purposes, outside of quite rare situations such as acute nausea and vomiting from chemotherapy, few indications exist for smoking cannabis. It is almost always preferable to eat cannabis and to maintain stable levels in the blood. If one regularly feels the immediate and psychoactive effects of the dose, it is too high.

Cultural and social attitudes about cannabis tend to be extreme. Some colleagues will never consider it a medicine until it is approved by

---

[18] Rotchford, JK, *Medical Cannabis - The Initial Medical Consultation*, Published through Amazon.com 2018

the FDA. Nonetheless, many effective and useful medications exist and have been used successfully throughout time well before there was ever an FDA. Controversy remains as well regarding dosing and the proper percentages of THC and CBDs in cannabis products. Aside from the advice to consume at a dose under which one feels it, and the importance of stable levels, particularly when using it long term for a chronic condition, a trial and error approach to dosing and concentrations is indicated.

Appendix—Publications / Resources

NOTE: *Purchasers of this book are invited to download a PDF online copy of the book with clickable links at DrRotchford.com/guide. The citatioons listed below, which do not show links, have links online.*

Publications—Recommended by Dr. Rotchford

A host of references are available online. I suggest "Google Scholar" and keyword searches to include: *methadone maintenance, opioid dependence,* and *opioid treatment.* Also do searches under the authors MJ Kreek, KL Sees, J. Kakko and look for related articles.

National Alliance of Advocates for Buprenorphine Treatment (NAABT) is an organization committed to promoting buprenorphine use in opiate dependency.

Substance Abuse and Mental Health Services Administration (SAMHSA)

American Society of Addictive Medicine is for physicians specializing in addiction medicine.

Role of Maintenance Treatment in Opioid Dependence—this a scholarly review of the essential need for Medication Assisted Treatment (MAT) in the care of opioid use disorders.

Methadone Maintenance vs 180-Day Psychosocially Enriched Detoxification for Treatment of Opioid Dependence A Randomized Controlled Trial, Karen L. Sees, DO; Kevin L. Delucchi, PhD; Carmen Masson, PhD; Amy Rosen, PsyD; H. Westley Clark, MD; Helen Robillard, RN, MSN, MA; Peter Banys, MD; Sharon M. Hall, PhD; *JAMA.* 2000;283:1303-1310.

Treatment for Opioid Dependence: Quality and Access; Bruce J. Rounsaville and Thomas R. Kosten; *JAMA*. 2000;283(10):1337-1339.

Provision of Methadone Treatment in Primary Care Medical Practices: Review of the Scottish Experience and Implications for US Policy; Michael Weinrich and Mary Stuart; *JAMA*. 2000;283(10):1343-1348.

1-year retention and social function after buprenorphine-assisted relapse prevention treatment for heroin dependence in Sweden: a randomised, placebo-controlled study; J Kakko, KD Svanborg, MJ Kreek, M Heilig - The Lancet, 2003 - Elsevier

Buprenorphine maintenance versus placebo or methadone maintenance for opioid dependence (A Cochrane Review) RP Mattick, J Kimber, C Breen, et al 2008 The link will take you to a reprint of a Cochrane review, prepared and maintained by The Cochrane Collaboration.

Handouts/References—On All Forms of SUDs

DrRotchford.com website provides links to articles, books, videos and other resources written by or compiled by Dr. Rotchford. Topics are varied but most often related to pain management or substance use disorders. Access the library at DrRotchford.com/handouts/.

Rotchford JK (2017) "Cultural Factors within the United States Promote Substance Use Disorders: A Helpful Perspective for Responding to the Opioid Misuse Epidemic." MOJ Addict Med Ther 4(1): 00069. DOI: 10.15406/mojamt.2017.04.00069

Websites—Hosted by Dr. Rotchford

DrRotchford.com— about Dr. Rotchford and his specialized practice.

Opioid Docs.com—Helpful access to national websites

[NOTE: All websites are accessible by smartphones and tablets]

Videos—Produced by Dr. Rotchford

Clinical Topics on Opioid Addiction For Addicts, Friends and Family by Dr. Rotchford.

To access videos go to DrRotchford.info

Session 1—Introduction to Basic Tools 9:23 min.
Session 2—Facing Dilemmas in Opioid Addiction 6:57min.
Session 3—Basic Tools in Opioid Addiction 5:46 min.
Session 4—How is Cutting Oneself Similar to Opioid Addiction? 12
Session 5—Shame and Blame 7:33 min.
Session 6—Medications for Opioid Addictions 4:09 min.
Session 7—Comorbid Conditions 7:10 min.
Session 8—1 2 3 of Recovery Help 11:18 min.
Session 9—Probuphine as an Option for Opioid Use Disorders 3:16
Session 10—You Can't Always Get What You Want 4:20 min.
Session 11—Naltrexone Use in Opioid Use Disorders 8:09 min.
Session 12—Playing Basketball: Opioid Use Disorders 4:38 min.

APPs—Developed by Dr. Rotchford

Opioid Doc.com—online and mobile access to helpful resources

OverdoseAPP.com—APP with practical help for overdose event

Other Publications by J. Kimber Rotchford, M.D.

Available online at www.DrRotchford.com under handouts tab

Addiction & Brain Health
What Promotes Recovery from Addictions
Brain Health 101
Help for Family Members
Trust—Making It a Non-Issue
PTSD—A Primer for Patients
Quitters Guide to Recovery from Marijuana and other Addictions
Self-Medicating
Medical Use of Addictive Substances

Pain Management
Review of Opiate Dependence in Pain Patients on Chronic Opioid Agonist Therapy (COAT)
Syllabus – Basics of Chronic Pain and Its Management
"The OPAS Experience," article in *Pain Practitioner*
Neuropathies—A Brief Overview
Managing Acute Pain in Patients on Buprenorphine
Managing Acute Pain in Patients Prescribed Methadone

Medications
Agonist Therapy—Buprenorphine and Methadone Therapy
Buprenorphine Patient Syllabus
Ketamine and Low Dose Therapy for Pain
Naltrexone to Treat Opiate Addiction
Probuphine—Game Changer for Opioid Use Disorders

Adjunctive Care
ACUPUNCTURE—A Brief Introduction
Medical Cannabis (Marijuana)—A Physician's Experience
Anxiety—A Discussion
Anger Issues in Those With Pain or Addiction Concerns
Grief and Grieving

About the Author

J. Kimber Rotchford, M.D., M.P.H has longstanding expertise in treating out-patients who suffer from chronic pain, addictions, and related disorders. Dr. Rotchford is among the earliest pain management specialists certified by the American Academy of Integrative Pain Management. Since 1981, he has emphasized and implemented integrative approaches to pain management.

His enduring interest and expertise in pain management led Dr. Rotchford to become a specialist in addiction medicine. He is one of the first physicians to be board certified in addiction medicine through the American Board of Addiction Medicine. He is the author of professional publications related to pain management and addiction medicine.

Dr. Rotchford is passionate about finding effective and practical solutions for pain management as well as for the opioid crisis. He has a strong background in public health and is a longstanding Fellow of the American College of Preventive Medicine. A native of Washington, he is a graduate of the University of Washington's School of Medicine and School of Public Health. The University of Washington has a noteworthy history of leadership and expertise in both chronic pain management and public health. He has also studied, worked, and taught internationally.

Recognized for his compassion and his expertise in the treatment of chronic pain and opioid use disorders, Dr. Rotchford has practiced for his entire clinical career in small towns in Washington State. First, he served patients on Washington's Pacific coast. For the past 25 years, he has practiced medicine in Port Townsend on the state's Olympic Peninsula.

Dr. Rotchford's full curriculum vitae is online at www.OPAS.us/resume

Acknowledgements: Dr. Rotchford wants to thank Ms. Andie Mitchell for her editing suggestions which complemented the professional services and encouragement of Mr. Dan Youra, without whom, this book would have never happened.

About the Editors

Dan Youra is the publisher and editor of books and magazines. He learned his skills as editor of *Current Thought on Peace and War*, published at the United Nations in New York. He is chairman of the board of directors for JC MASH free clinic in Port Townsend, Washington.

Andie Mitchell is a freelance writer and editor. She also works in garden restoration and design. She lives in Port Townsend, WA with her family.

Opidemic—A Public Health Epidemic

Olympas Medical Services
J. Kimber Rotchford, M.D., M.P.H.

Olympas Pain and Addiction Services Clinic
1136 Water St. Suite 107
Port Townsend, WA 98368

www.OPAS.us
staff@OPAS.us

www.ingramcontent.com/pod-product-compliance
Lightning Source LLC
Chambersburg PA
CBHW062220220526
45471CB00009B/3276